Recipes for Natural Beauty

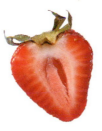

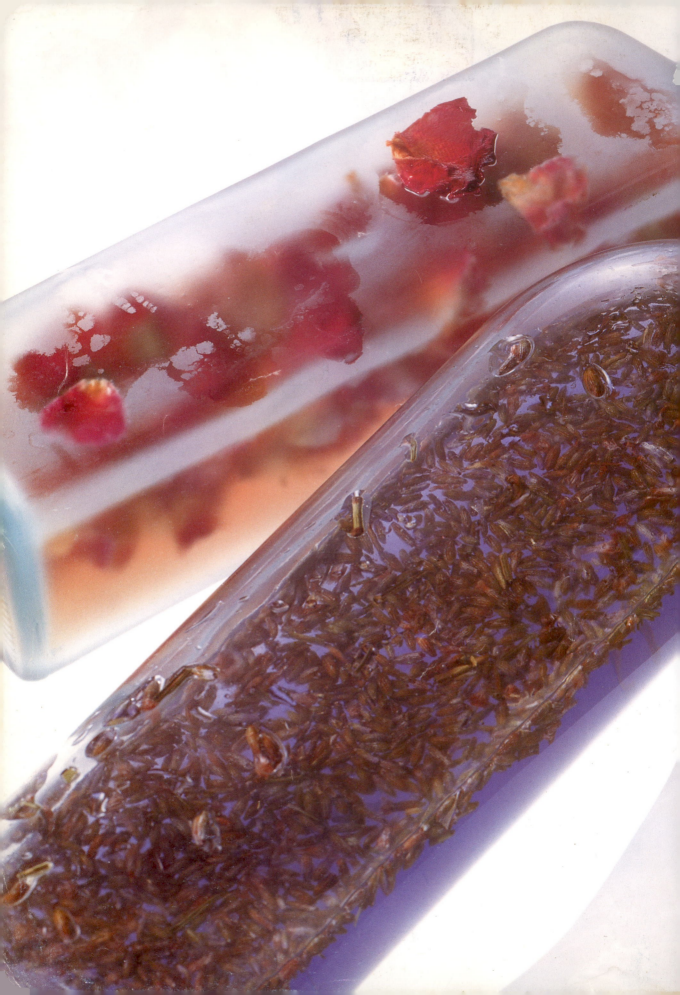

Recipes for
Natural Beauty

Katie Spiers

Facts On File, Inc.

Recipes for Natural Beauty

Copyright © 1998 by Quarto Inc.

Library of Congress Cataloging-in-Publication Data

Spiers, Katie.
Recipes for natural beauty: 100 homemade treatments for natural
beauty / by Katie Spiers.
p. cm.
Includes index.
ISBN 0-8160-3828-7
1. Beauty, Personal. 2. Skin—Care and hygiene. 3. Hair—Care
and hygiene. 4. Herbal cosmetics. 1. Title.
RA778.S732 1998   98-9367
646.7 2—dc21

For information contact:
Facts On File, Inc.
11 Penn Plaza
New York NY 10001

Facts On File books are available at special discounts when purchased in bulk
quantities for businesses, associations, institutions or sales promotions. Please
call our Special Sales Department in New York at (212) 967-8800
or (800) 322-8755.

You can find Facts On File on the World Wide Web at
http://www.factsonfile.com

This book was designed and produced by
Quarto Publishing plc
6 Blundell Street
London N7 9BH

Project editor Anne Hildyard
Art editor Luise Roberts
Photographer Will White
Editor Carole Clements
Art director Moira Clinch

10 9 8 7 6 5 4 3 2 1

This book is printed on acid-free paper.
Typeset by CST Typesetters, Eastbourne

Printed by Leefung–Asco Printers Ltd, China

Manufactured by Universal Graphics Pte Ltd, Singapore

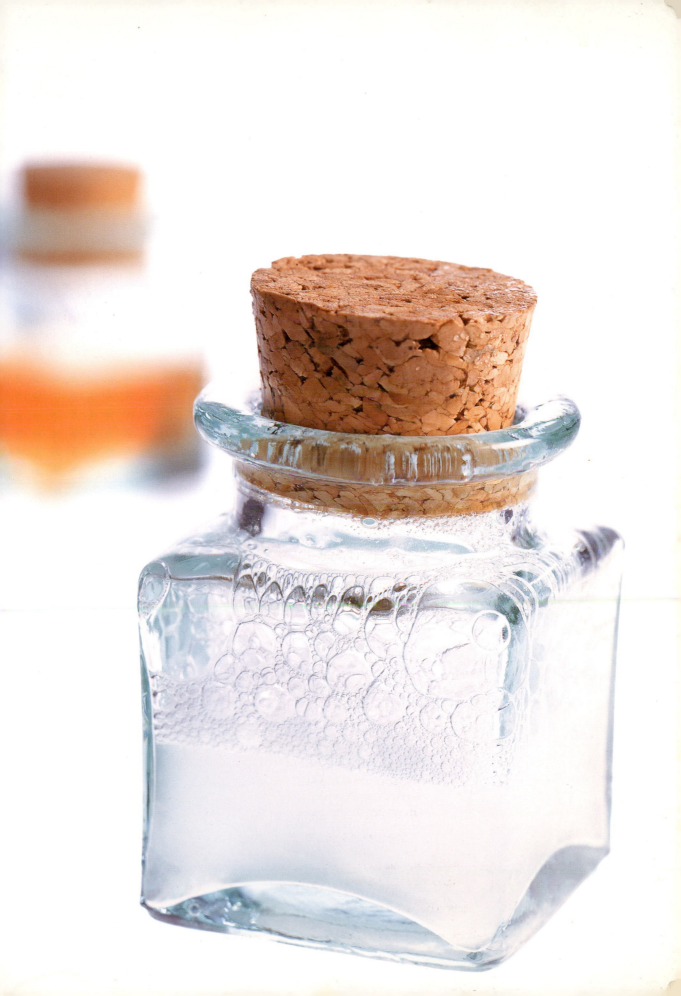

FOREWORD

"True radiant beauty comes from within." This statement from the text of this book establishes the link that makes the work so valuable. In fact, this understanding makes it possible for the author to produce a multi-dimensional book that truly fills a gap in today's literature of health. This concise volume brings together nutrition, attitudes, emotional tone, self-confidence and spiritual awareness and relates them to the freshness and vitality that we recognize as beauty.

The skin as it has been created for us is a marvelous work of art. It is also a vital organ, since when enough of it is taken away, as with an extensive burn, we perish. The skin and the various glands (for sweat and oil) and appendages (such as hair and nails) associated with it perform a multitude of essential functions. Among these we can list temperature regulation; the balance of water, salts, acids and bases; protection against physical, chemical and microbial injury; detection of a wide variety of noxious stimuli; and the provision of an elastic covering that accommodates the movements of the underlying structures. In fact, all of these functions are connected to and are reflections of internal processes that are vital to life. And we must also remind ourselves how profoundly the attractiveness of the skin, hair, nails, eyes and mouth affects all of our social and intimate interactions.

It is important that the way we treat these accessible parts of the body enhance the various connections I have mentioned, rather than detract from them in any way. Thus, all the ingredients for the many recipes included in this volume should be from pure natural sources, as indeed they are. The instructions for the preparation and use of the recipes included should be simple and straightforward, thus making the materials completely accessible to the user, and so, to a remarkable degree, they are. The information contained herein should be, and is, obtained from reliable sources that reflect at least generations of experience in its use, plus an adequate record of safety and efficacy.

Those who peruse this book will find elements of a number of recognized disciplines, including herbal therapy, aromatherapy and therapeutic massage, as well as techniques of selection, mixing and application that derive from many cultures and parts of the globe. Diet and lifestyle considerations are included, which give a good balance to the more local treatments that are described. In addition, upon careful reading of the text, I find nothing in its pages that is medically unsound.

I heartily recommend "Recipes for Natural Beauty" to those who are seeking wellness in body, mind, emotions and spirit, as reflected externally by a vibrant aura and an attractive glow of health.

Peter Albright, M.D.

CONTENTS

INTRODUCTION

By making your own cosmetics you have absolute control over which ingredients are used and how fresh they are. The idea that cosmetics can be individually made to suit specific needs and skin types means you will never be without a preparation that meets your needs perfectly. As you gain confidence with making up these preparations, you will find yourself experimenting with different ingredients and making a true art out of creating your own beauty preparations.

Remember that beauty comes from within, both literally and metaphorically. You need to look after your system by eating well and sleeping and exercising enough.

Making up recipes as you need them means you are being kinder to the environment as well as your pocket. All ingredients in this book are fairly inexpensive, readily available and have the benefit of natural enzyme action. They are easy to prepare and apply.

I hope that you will have as much fun making and using these cosmetics as I have.

STORAGE

The way you store your preparations is important because incorrect handling can ruin the effectiveness, and even cause damage to your skin. Try to use dark glass or plastic bottles and jars, which seal up well. You want to avoid too much oxygen and sunlight getting to your cosmetics. Keep fresh preparations in a cool place, preferably the refrigerator, especially those containing fruit or vegetables. Most of the recipes in this book contain natural preservatives.

preservatives

Essential oils
Tea tree, thyme and eucalyptus oil

Acids
Lemon juice and vinegar

Alcohols
Vodka, brandy and witch hazel

When using alcohols in a recipe, vodka is the best as it has little fragrance and is very strong. Never use preparations that look moldy or stale.

BASIC TECHNIQUES

The following methods will provide you with the basic techniques that are used frequently when making the recipes in this book. They describe in greater detail the processes used for the preparation of the recipe components together with some useful tips and hints on preparing, measuring and mixing ingredients. Although quantities in the recipes are not critical, it is best to be guided by the amounts stated.

getting started

Preparing and blending fruits and vegetables for application on the skin

Always use fresh fruit wherever possible. Wait until all the other ingredients are assembled before cutting; this keeps the potent enzymes as fresh as possible.

Measuring

Be guided by the ingredients and techniques specified in the recipes, but please remember you do not have to be too rigid about this. Ingredients vary from place to place, especially where they are natural, so be flexible and use your intuition.

How to mix up oils for use in aromatherapy

Always drop essential oils being added to a base oil into the center of the oil and not down the side of the bottle or jar. Avoid the dropper touching the bottle or jar. To mix, seal the oil and shake gently, or rub the bottle between your palms quickly to warm the oil and mix the ingredients.

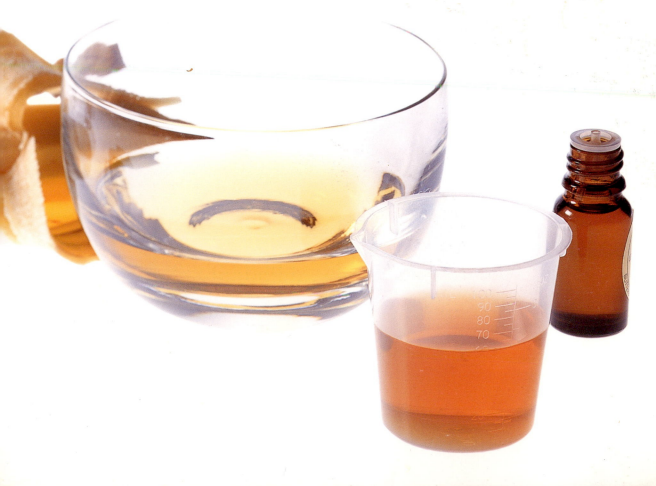

making basic ingredients

How to melt solid fats

This method provides a gentle heat source to safeguard delicate ingredients such as beeswax. It is often used by chefs to melt chocolate and it is sometimes known as the chocolate method.

1) Half-fill a small saucepan with water.

2) Heat the water until it is simmering and place a heatproof bowl of glass, ceramic or plastic over the water, resting the bowl on the sides of the pan so the bottom of the bowl does not touch the surface of the water.

3) Place the ingredient to be heated in the bowl over the water. Do this immediately or the empty bowl may become too hot and could crack.

4) Heat the ingredient, keeping the water underneath simmering gently. Do not allow it to boil.

To blend a lotion or cream

When blending an oil or tincture into a base cream, fold it in gently. Make sure the oil is very evenly distributed and that a certain amount of air is kept in the lotion. Do not pack it too tightly in a bottle or jar.

How to make an infusion

Herbs need to be infused for enough time to extract the goodness, but not so much they denature or become soggy. A rough guide is approximately ten minutes infusing for a normal herb and fifteen minutes for a root or bark. The recipe will usually tell you how long to infuse your herb.

1) Place the herb in the quantity specified in the recipe in the bottom of a bowl or mug. Use a bowl that can withstand heat; avoid glass unless it is heatproof (e.g.: Pyrex).

2) Pour over the water; for most recipes use about 2 cups (480 ml), or as specified. Make sure the water has boiled, but use just off the boil.

3) Allow the herb to infuse for the specified amount of time, then strain the infused liquid. Discard the used herb.

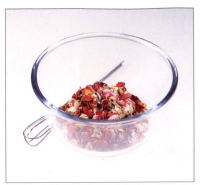
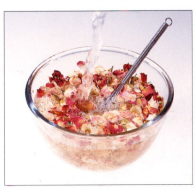

To make a tincture

This is a complicated process that usually involves distillation equipment. If you want to make your own tinctures, I suggest you find a good book that outlines the various methods of distillation and seeping. Tinctures are fairly inexpensive and easy to buy. Alternatively, you may wish to try the less effective seeping method. Place the herbs to be used in a bowl with alcohol (brandy is by far the best, as you need a mild smelling dark alcohol for tinctures) and allow to stand in a warm place for at least forty eight hours. Strain and discard the herb, and bottle the mild tincture.

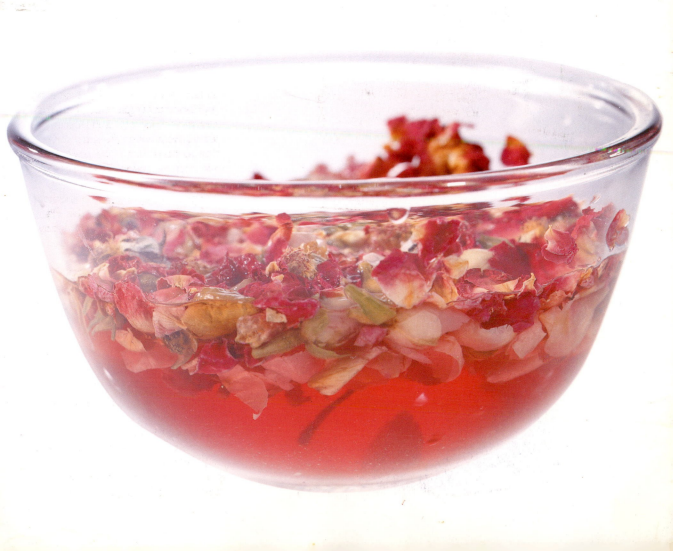

INGREDIENTS

Alcohol

An antiseptic astringent, it tightens the skin and acts as a natural preservative. Brandy is best for use in tinctures; vodka is best in most other cases, as it has the least fragrance and is very strong.

Base oil

A bland non-fragranced oil that moisturizes the skin.

Baking soda (bicarbonate of soda)

A white powder that foams slightly in water and eventually dissolves. Highly cleansing.

Aloe vera gel

A jelly-like material extracted from aloe vera, a succulent plant that is cooling and soothing.

Emollient

Soothes and softens the skin.

Cocoa butter
A solid fat that gives body to creams and lotions and softens the skin.

Coconut oil
A fat derived from the coconut (one of the few vegetarian fats), it melts at body temperature.

Beeswax
Secreted by bees to build the walls of their cells, it softens the skin and does not clog pores.

terms and ingredients

Base dispersing oil
A bland base oil that disperses in water, usually used to make bath preparations, it is readily available from health stores.

Essential oil
Oil from plants or fruits in a very strong, concentrated form.

Lanolin
A moisturizing oil obtained from sheep's wool.

Organic
Organic produce is grown without the use of pesticides and other chemical products. The average non-organic strawberry has been sprayed 22 times before it reaches you. Always try to buy organic produce.

Kaolin
A type of clay used in making porcelain or china and also for medical purposes, it helps to draw impurities from the skin.

Honey
There are many different types of honey. Looser consistency honeys, such as acacia and Greek, are probably the best to use in cosmetics.

Green clay
A heavy, mineral-rich clay that helps draw impurities from the skin.

Glycerin
Made from petroleum, this is a mineral-based skin softener.

Infusion
A mixture of herbs and water that has been allowed to seep or soak and then is strained. The liquid remaining is the infusion.

Tincture
An alcohol solution of an herb.

Herbs
Can be used dried or fresh, fresh are better though, and you may wish to grow your own. It is important to use fresh herbs when the herb itself is an ingredient and not just the liquor from a herb. Fresh herbs are generally needed in slightly larger quantities than dried as the dried variety is more potent.

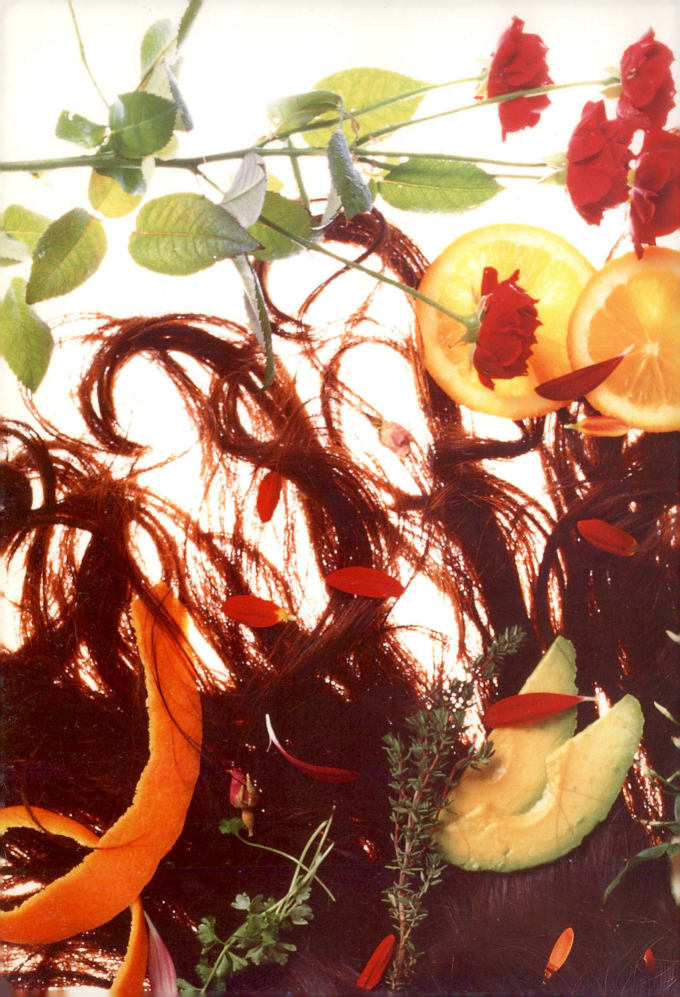

RECIPES

SKIN

Everyone's skin is different, and the quality of your skin will depend very much on a range of factors including how well you take care of it, the quality of the air it is exposed to both long and short term, your lifestyle, diet and, unfortunately, your age. One thing skin quality rarely depends on is the amount of money you spend on cosmetics. Often the best skin care regime is simple but well thought out and designed to suit your needs. Fresh, carefully made beauty products can be as good as or better than commercial products. This is because you have absolute control over what goes into preparations you make and can avoid preservatives or any ingredients that do not suit you personally. The live cultures and invigorating enzymes in fresh cosmetics make them unbeatable for bringing life and vitality to your skin.

There are, of course, many natural preparations on the market, but although they are a preferable choice to synthetic or mineral based cosmetics, many of them include hidden ingredients. The recipes here are all wholesome and totally pure, for wholesome and pure skin!

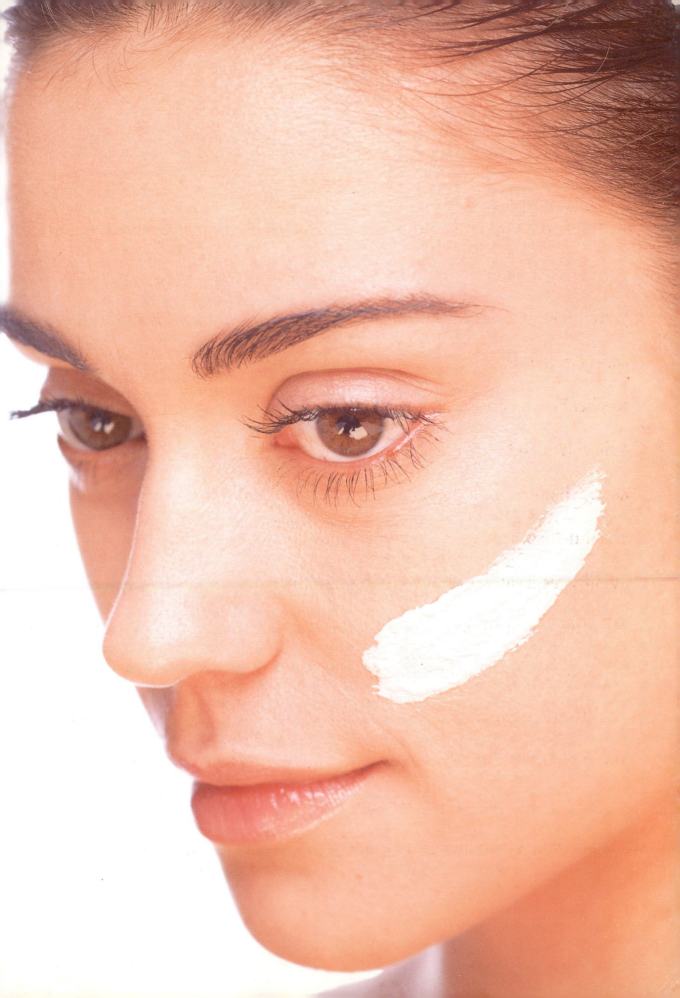

SKIN TYPE

There is a very simple test for identifying your skin type. Simply peel a single-ply sheet from a tissue and gently press it to your face. When you remove the tissue if you see a greasy residue you have oily skin; no residue indicates dry skin. Try testing patches of your skin to see if it varies from area to area; most skins do.

different skin types

NORMAL SKIN

This is the type of skin we all aspire to have but few of us are blessed with. Skin naturally is healthy and vibrant (just look at the complexions of young children), but time and modern living take their toll. A good skin care routine helps to redevelop the natural balance we all once had.

Grapefruit and Glycerin Mask

Glycerin is an emollient (lubricant). Combined with grapefruit for cleansing and toning, it creates a face mask that cleanses, rehydrates and tightens the skin.

Ingredients

2 tbsp (30 ml) liquid glycerin

1 tbsp (15 ml) coarsely grated grapefruit peel

2 tsp (10 ml) fresh grapefruit juice (optional)

2 drops grapefruit essential oil

To make

Mix the glycerin with the grapefruit peel. If the mixture is very sticky, either heat the glycerin slightly by adding a teaspoon of boiling water or add some grapefruit juice. Add the essential oil and mix thoroughly until it forms a thick paste. Keeps for up to two weeks in the refrigerator.

To use

Apply evenly over the skin, avoiding the eye area. If using direct from the refrigerator, allow to warm slightly or the consistency will be too thick — it should be like honey. Leave on for at least twenty minutes and rinse, using the grapefruit peel to rub the skin and gently exfoliate.

OILY SKIN

Teenagers often suffer with this skin type, which can lead to blemishes and acne. If we work too hard to strip the natural oil (sebum), a natural counteraction will occur and more oil will be produced. This condition is known as seborrhea.

Gentle cleansing, regular steaming and an occasional deep-working face mask is the best way to treat this type of skin.

Aloe Vera and Rose Hip Mask

Aloe vera has healing properties for pimples and it also moisturizes and cleanses. If you have an aloe plant you can actually cut a frond and squeeze a small amount of juice from it to apply to the skin. Rose hip is astringent and a light cleanser.

Ingredients

1 tbsp (15 ml) strong rose hip infusion

4 tbsp (60 ml) aloe vera gel (make sure it is pure)

2 drops rosemary essential oil

To make

Make up the rose hip infusion (see page 13). Gradually stir the infusion into the aloe vera gel. You are looking for the consistency of loose gel—you may not need all the infusion. Then add the essential oil (for stimulating and antiseptic properties) and mix again thoroughly.

To use

This gel should be applied cold direct from the refrigerator. The coolness will have an excellent tonic effect and it feels wonderful when it slides onto the skin. You should remove when it has warmed to the skin; this mask will not dry much.

DRY SKIN

Dry skin is often flaky and can crack and become extremely uncomfortable. Psoriasis and eczema are severe forms of dry skin. I would try to avoid the steroid creams that you may be prescribed by your doctor for such conditions. Your body can develop a kind of immunity to these so the strength has to be increased and eventually they may become totally ineffective.

Banana and Honey Rehydrator

Nourishing banana provides intense moisture and gives a delicious rich fragrance to this mask. Honey is soothing and nourishing.

Ingredients

1 ripe banana

2 tbsp (30 ml) acacia honey

1 tbsp (15 ml) fresh live natural yogurt

To make

Mash the banana with a fork, add other ingredients and mix thoroughly. If you have a blender, use it! Make sure the honey is warm enough to disperse through the other ingredients. Honey should be kept at room temperature; it will crystallize in the refrigerator.

To use

Apply in generous quantities over the face and neck. Do not apply in a steamy bath because it will slide off! Allow to dry (15 minutes or so) and remove. You can also use this preparation over sluggish areas such as thighs.

CLEANSING

Cleansing the skin is perhaps the most important part of skin care. Throughout the day the skin picks up a huge amount of dirt and pollution, especially if you live in a city. It is very important not to leave this grime on the face overnight. Traditionally soap and water was used as a cleanser; however, we now know that the pH of soap can strip the skin and leave it dry and tight. Deep cleansing can occur when the face is steamed or warmed and the pores of the skin open. Usually a deep cleansing once or twice a week is enough. Do not deep cleanse the day before a special occasion, as drawing out impurities from the skin in this way can lead to blemishes, so allow a couple of days for the skin to settle.

step-by-step cleansing

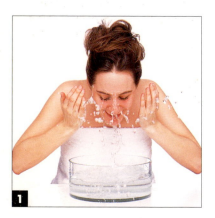

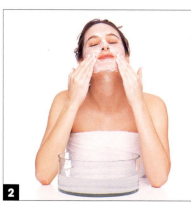

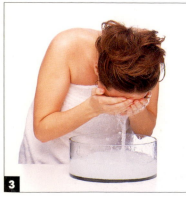

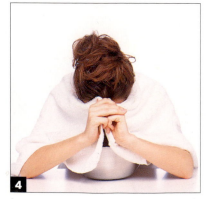

1) If you have long hair keep it off your face with a headband. Wash your hands in warm water. Moisten your face using either a sponge or face cloth, or with your hands. If you use a sponge, I suggest using a natural sponge. Make sure you rinse it well after use, as damp sponges and face cloths are breeding grounds for germs.

2) Lather the face using one of the cleansers appropriate to your skin type. Now would be a good time to gently massage the facial muscles (see the massage section). Try to avoid getting soap in your eyes.

3) Rinse your face thoroughly. If you wish to steam the face now is the time to do so.

4) Fill a bowl with hot water and, using a towel to keep the steam and heat in, hold your face over the bowl for a few minutes. Removing all traces of cleanser from the face is very important and this is completed with the next stage of the skin care routine, toning.

Jojoba Two-in-One Cleanser and Moisturizer

For dry or normal skin, this simple mixture of jojoba and grapeseed oils produces a deep cleansing, yet nondrying, intense moisturizer.

Ingredients

2 tbsp (30 ml) jojoba oil

2 tsp (10 ml) grapeseed oil

1 drop geranium essential oil

To make

Combine all ingredients in a small bottle. Close the lid tightly and shake to mix the oils well.

To use

This preparation should be applied with a cotton ball and smoothed lightly on the skin. Do not apply too much or it will be clogging. Use gentle strokes to apply and remove, rubbing any excess oil into the skin for extra moisturizing.

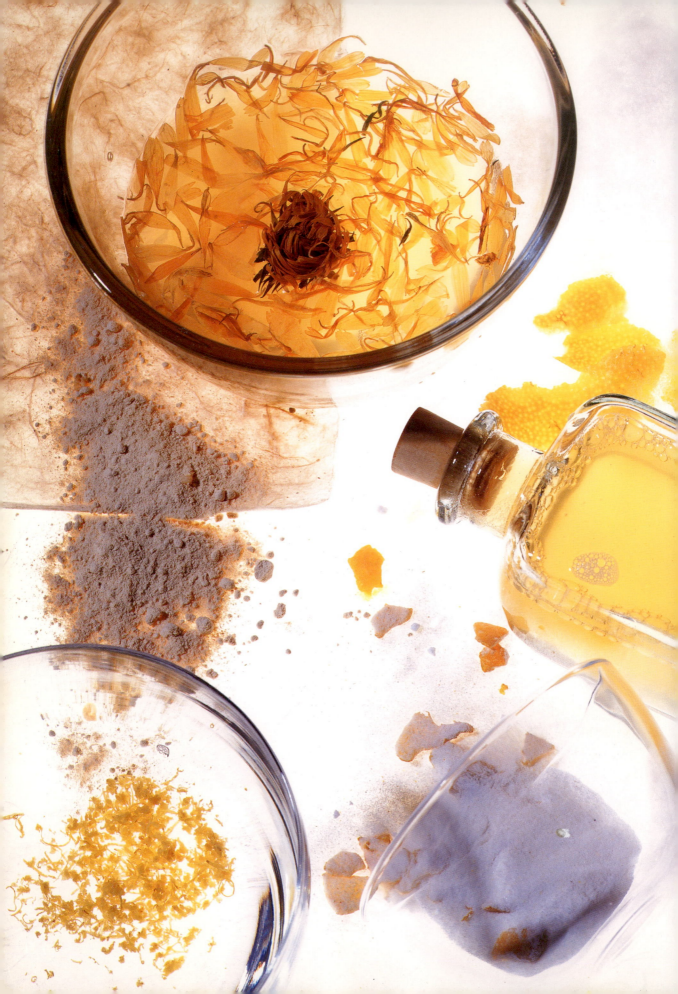

cleansing

Baking Soda Scrub

This mix of rice grains (used in Japan for cleansing and smoothing the skin) and baking soda, renowned for its mildly abrasive cleaning properties, is particularly suitable for oily skin.

Ingredients

2 tbsp (30 ml) baking soda

2 tbsp (30 ml) ground rice
(you can buy it ground, or grind it yourself in a small coffee grinder)

1 tsp (5 ml) soap crystals (optional)

1 tsp (5 ml) finely grated lemon peel

To make

All ingredients in this recipe are dry so they may be mixed together and stored for a fairly long time (baking soda is a natural preservative). Fresh lemon peel is best, but if you prefer you can buy the dried variety in herb and spice shops. If you cannot obtain soap crystals they may be left out, but the scrub will not lather.

To use

The rough texture of this scrub means it will remove dead skin cells, leaving you with a fresh and clean skin. Apply in small handfuls and vigorously rub into areas of the face until the soap lathers up. Dry your face with a soft towel and gently apply moisturizer if required.

Orange Sorbet Hot Weather Cleanser

Orange flower water and petitgrain make a deliciously smelling, fresh, light cleanser. Great for use in very hot weather to leave the skin feeling clear and bright. (Petitgrain is a fragrant essential oil derived from the leaves and branches of trees of the *Citrus* genus.)

Ingredients

4 tbsp (60 ml) orange flower water

5 drops petitgrain essential oil

2 tsp (10 ml) calendula petals

1 pinch orris root (optional)

To make

Mix all the ingredients together in a bottle. If you wish the cleanser to keep longer, add the orris root as a preservative. The calendula flowers look really pretty and soften in the water, releasing cleansing properties. They are renowned as a cleanser in the form of calendula applications.

To use

Apply with cotton balls, or alternatively, splash on the face and neck as a light fragrance. I carry this preparation in my handbag in the summer and use it throughout the day. Avoid getting in the eyes, as the alcohol base from the orange flower water will sting.

TONING

Toning is a very simple process, its main action to remove any remaining traces of cleanser. It tightens the skin in preparation for moisturizing. If you have steamed your face after cleansing, toning tightens up the pores of the skin. This is important before you apply makeup. Water itself is the most natural toner. Use lukewarm or more revitalizing cold water, but avoid hot water, which can damage the cells of the facial skin.

toner recipes to suit your skin type

Rose and Mallow Spritzer

For dry skin, this has a rose water base with a moisture inducing mallow infusion.

Ingredients

4 tbsp (60 ml) rose water	
2 tbsp (30 ml) mallow infusion	
2 tbsp (30 ml) vodka	
2 tsp (10 ml) rose petals	
1 drop rose essential oil (optional)	

To make

See page 15 for instructions for making up the mallow infusion. Mallow is a very gentle herb with a lovely soft fragrance. Do not leave to infuse for too long, however, or it becomes bitter. Mix the rose water and mallow infusion with the vodka, which acts as a preservative. The rose petals and oil are not essential but do give the toner a slightly more luxurious feel. Rose oil can be very expensive, but it is worth the investment.

To use

The best way to apply this toner is to put it into a spray-top bottle. Plastic atomizers can be bought cheaply from garden centers. Spraying this fine mist over your face is cooling and tightens the skin. It's great for sunny days straight from the refrigerator.

Lemon Witch Hazel Toner

The freshest lemon juice in an alcohol base will blot away excess oil and grime from oily skin.

Ingredients

2 tbsp (30 ml) vodka	
2 tbsp (30 ml) fresh lemon juice	
1 tsp (5 ml) witch hazel	
1 tbsp (15 ml) water	

To make

Mix all the ingredients thoroughly. It is important that the lemon juice is freshly squeezed, as the bottled variety has antioxidizing chemicals in it that are not pure enough for application on the face.

To use

This toner is quite strong in its astringent (oil-removing) effect. To moderate it, I suggest either not including the alcohol, in which case it will not last as long because alcohol is a good preservative, or simply not using this preparation every day. Apply in the usual way and don't leave on the skin for too long. Rinse off with warm water. Do not apply to broken skin—it will sting!

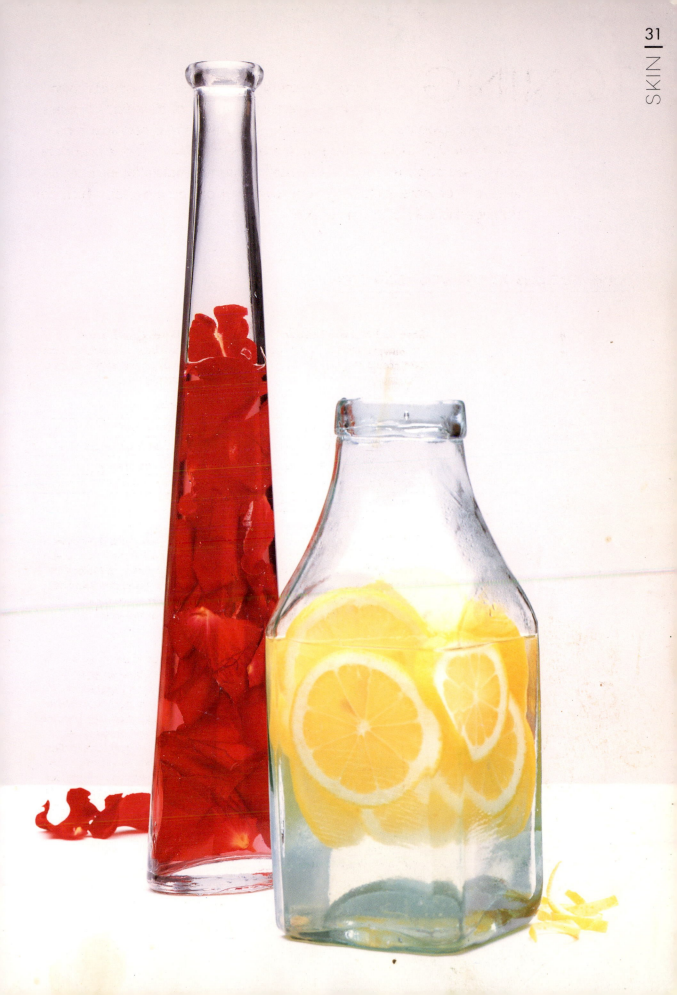

toning

Three Flower Cleanser

A wonderful combination of three traditional flower waters, gentle and soothing, this cleanser was used in Victorian times. Simple yet effective.

Ingredients

2 tbsp (30 ml) witch hazel

2 tbsp (30 ml) rose water

2 tbsp (30 ml) elderflower water

To make

Simply place all the ingredients in a bottle and mix together thoroughly.

To use

Apply as a normal toner. Especially good as a two-in-one, this toner will also cleanse the skin if applied with cotton balls. Witch hazel draws out impurities from the skin and is softened with the addition of elderflower to soothe and calm the skin. Rose water adds its delicious fragrance.

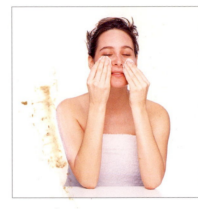

Camomile Toner

For sensitive skin, this soothing and cooling toner is a good after-sun treatment.

Ingredients

2 tbsp (30 ml) camomile infusion (see page 13)

1–2 drops camomile essential oil

2 tbsp (30 ml) water

1 tsp (5 ml) calendula petals

To make

Mix all the ingredients. You may either add the flowers at the end, or add them to the camomile while it is infusing to gain more of their soothing properties. If your camomile oil is very high quality, use only one drop, as any more may be overpowering.

To use

Great straight from the refrigerator to cool irritated skin on a hot day. If sprayed straight onto the skin, it is a good, calming soother for sunburn or heat rash.

Grape Tonic

A bitter, alcohol-based toner, it leaves the skin tingling and rich in minerals.

Ingredients

2 tbsp (30 ml) grape juice

2 tbsp (30 ml) water

1 tsp (5 ml) Swedish bitters
    or 1 tsp (5 ml) milk thistle tincture

To make

If you have a juice extractor to make grape juice yourself do so, because including the skins of the grapes in this process will increase the antioxidant effect of this tonic, which is great news for your skin! Mix the ingredients together, adding the bitters or tincture to the juice and water bit by bit, until the liquid is a very pale brown (you may not need all). Do not add too much tincture as this will make the tonic too strong.

To use

Swedish bitters and milk thistle tincture are extremely good herbal mixtures for the skin, especially problem skins. (Try to find Swedish bitters, but if you cannot, milk thistle tincture has similar cleansing properties.) When taken internally they cleanse the liver (do not try without the supervision of a qualified practitioner). Applied to the skin they heal and restore. The best way to apply this tonic is to lightly spray on the face with an atomizer. Do not over use, as this recipe is fairly strong. Although the alcohol acts as a preservative, grapes are among the highest in sugar of all fruits so the shelf life of this tonic may not be as long as that of others.

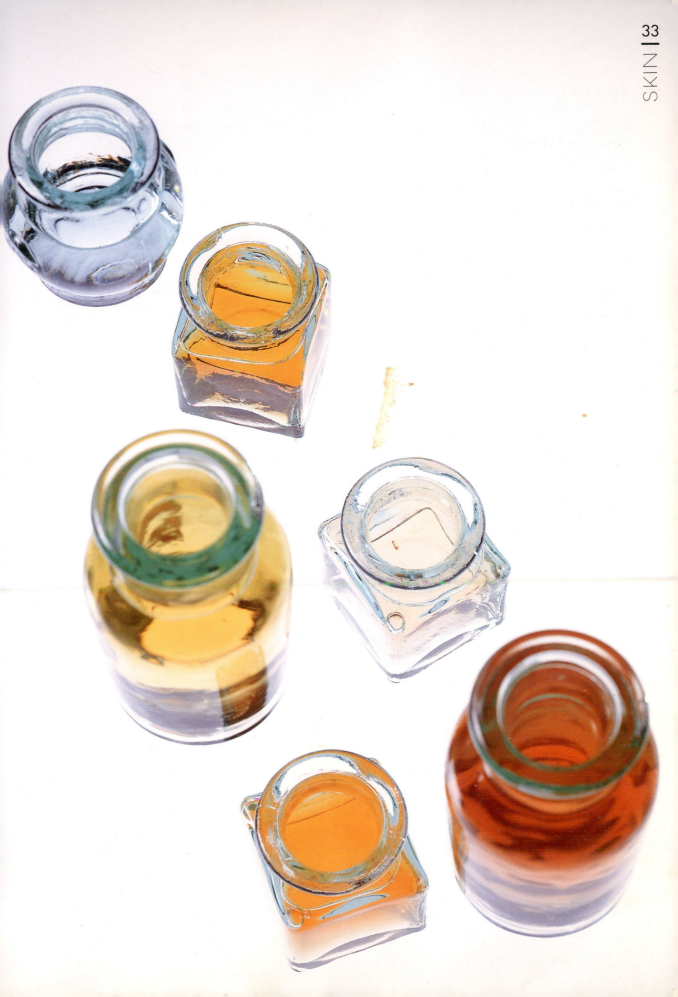

MOISTURIZING

It is very important to moisturize even skin that may seem oily, otherwise the body will produce too much natural oil (sebum), which clogs the pores and may lead to blemishes. It is a myth that only dry skins need moisturizing. However, if you do have oily skin use a light lotion rather than any heavier salve. The best time to moisturize is after toning. You may apply body lotion after a hot bath, when the pores are open, as more moisture is absorbed this way, but do not apply moisture to the face at this time, as it will feel clogged. Wait until the pores of the skin have closed a little before moisturizing the face or applying makeup.

recipes for moisturizers

Nourishing Orange Oil

Jojoba oil with the rich oil and fresh peel of orange is great for dry skin.

Ingredients

1 orange
2 tbsp (30 ml) jojoba oil
2 drops orange essential oil

To make

Make sure the orange is clean and organic. Using a vegetable peeler, remove the colored part of the skin without taking any of the white pith. Combine the oils in a bowl and place the orange peel in it. Leave to infuse at least twenty four hours. Do not refrigerate as this slows enzyme

action. Remove the peel and decant the oil into a storage bottle.

To use

This oil is fairly rich but very nourishing. It may be used to avoid stretch marks developing on the skin. Use in small quantities and massage deeply in to the skin. This oil is best

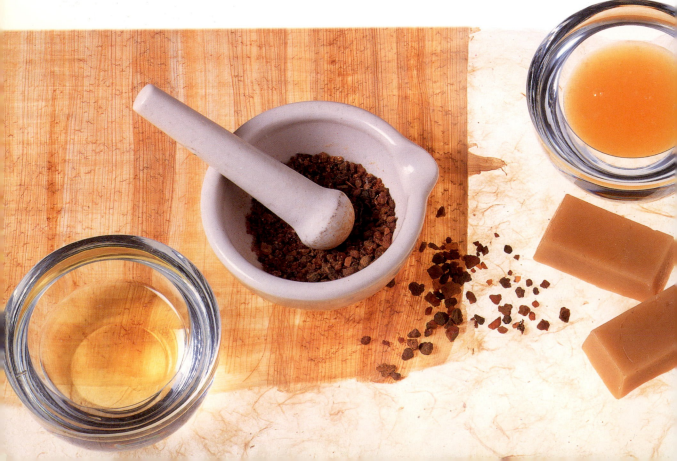

as a facial oil, but do not add too much essential oil or it will turn your face a very unhealthy looking orange!

Simple Honey Cream or Lotion

A good all-around base and medium moisturizer for normal skin, this contains beeswax and gentle acacia honey. It has an absolutely divine fragrance and leaves the skin silky smooth.

Ingredients

1 tbsp (15 ml) beeswax
1 tbsp (15 ml) acacia honey
2 tbsp (30 ml) base cream

To make

The beeswax needs heating. You can heat it carefully in a small bowl over a pan of lightly simmering water (this is known as the chocolate method—so called because chefs use it to melt chocolate, which is too delicate for the application of direct heat). In a small bowl (or blender container),

add the honey to the wax and beat together vigorously. You need to be quick at this stage to ensure complete dispersion before the wax solidifies, then add and mix in the base cream. The best way by far of mixing this in is in a blender, especially if you are using larger quantities.

If the cream is very sticky, use less honey. Acacia is the best honey to use but any type of runny honey will do.

To use

This cream will last a fairly long time, especially if it is thoroughly mixed. Apply in generous amounts to the face. For a lighter body lotion add more base cream.

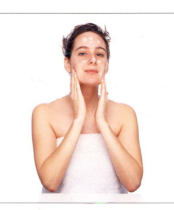

Myrrh Moisturizer

This light moisturizer for oily skin contains extract of natural myrrh resin. It reduces oil and has an excellent antifungal property. Myrrh moisturizer is great for treating problem skin conditions.

Ingredients

1 drop tea tree essential oil
4 tbsp (60 ml) base cream
1 tsp (5 ml) myrrh resin

To make

Mix the essential oil into the base cream, then add the resin and mix thoroughly. You may grind the resin to a very fine powder and include it in the application of the cream, but unless you have a powerful grinder this may make the cream gritty. The other alternative is to include the resin lumps in the cream but avoid applying them to the skin; they simply remain in the cream as a natural preservative and lend their healing properties to the preparation.

To use

Make sure the myrrh resin is very high quality and very clean. Myrrh sold for the purpose of incense burning will rarely be of a high enough standard. Apply the cream morning and evening to problem skin areas after cleansing and toning. Do not use every day on normal skins. May be made in a slightly stronger form to apply directly to blemishes or small problem areas.

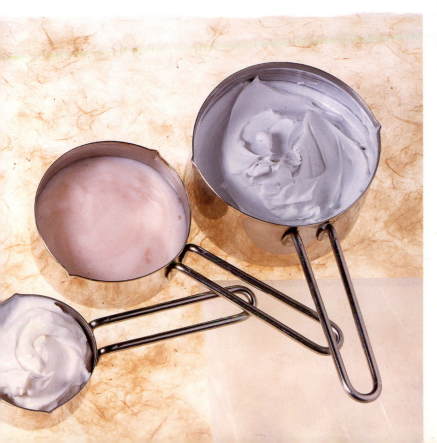

moisturizer and massage bar

Milk and Rosemary Moisturizer

Made with milk, this preparation is nourishing and luxurious, a variation on an ancient recipe.

Ingredients

4 tbsp (60 ml) whole milk

2 drops rosemary essential oil

2 sprigs fresh rosemary (optional)

To make

This is a moisturizing mix for a relaxing bath. Add the milk and essential oil to the bath. The milk helps the oil disperse, so give the water a good swish.

To use

If you wish, you can also wrap fresh rosemary in cheesecloth and make a giant "tea bag." Place this under the running water (you may wish to tie it to the faucet so it does remain under the running water). The infusion from these herbs in your bath is very luxurious. Use with or instead of the cream mixture.

Strawberry Moisture Bar

A solid, melt-in-the-hands moisture inducing bar, this is made with cocoa butter and beeswax.

Ingredients

2 tbsp (30 ml) beeswax

2 tbsp (30 ml) cocoa butter

1 tsp (5 ml) thick honey

3 strawberries

To make

Heat the beeswax and cocoa butter together in a bowl over a pan of lightly simmering water. Add the honey and mix vigorously. You will need a mold or small bowl for setting the bar. Line this with parchment paper, place the strawberries in the bottom of the mold, then pour the beeswax and cocoa butter mixture over the top. These quantities make a fairly small bar, but it does last, so you may wish to make up more. The key to this recipe is keeping the beeswax mixture very hot so it does not solidify while you are working with it. Once the bar is made, refrigerate at least overnight to harden, then remove from the mold and paper.

To use

The strawberries add fragrance and color; they need not be applied to the skin. Rub the bar between your hands to warm it for use, then rub into the skin, either as a moisturizer or as a massage bar. Do not let the whole bar get too warm or it will disintegrate.

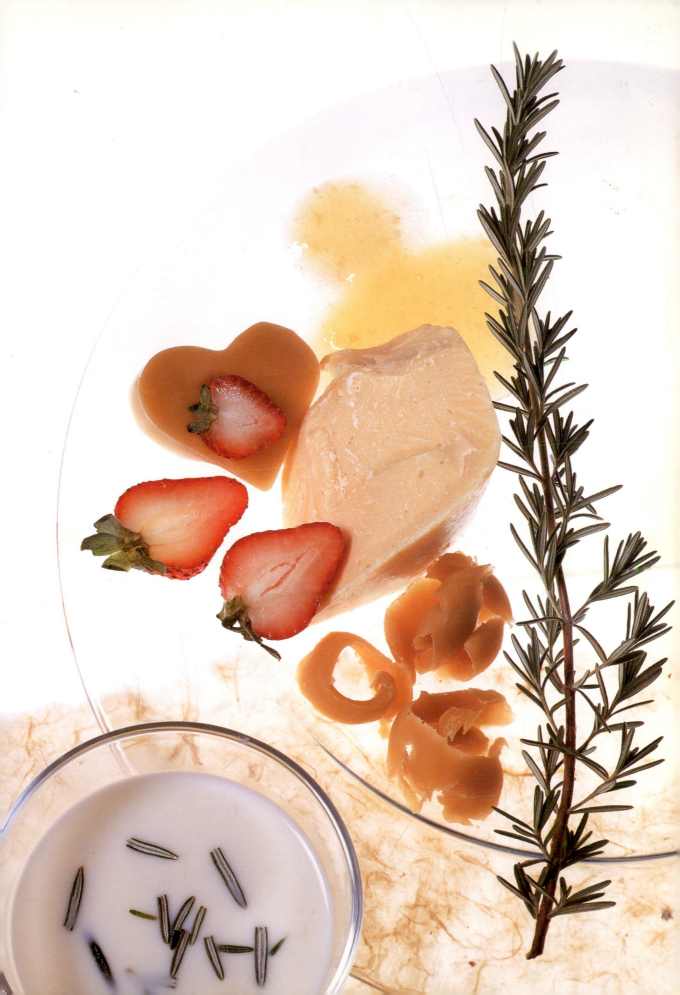

EXFOLIATORS

Exfoliation is the process of using a mildly abrasive agent on the skin to remove dead skin cells. Your skin will soon show the benefits of regular deep exfoliation. Exfoliation works by removing dead skin cells from the skin's surface. Our skin renews itself completely every month, so exfoliation will keep it smooth and clear. Exfoliating also cleanses skin and removes grime and buildup without stripping skin of natural sebum oil. To avoid this stripping, it is important not to exfoliate too often, which can be a temptation, especially if you are prone to pimples. Ideally, exfoliate no more than once a week.

skin smoothers

Bran and Oatmeal Scrub

As a once a week deep cleanser, oatmeal helps to break down the impurities while bran gently lifts them from the surface of the skin.

Ingredients

1 cup (240 ml) bran
1 cup (240 ml) oatmeal
2 tbsp (30 ml) whole milk

To make

Mix the bran and oatmeal together and add the milk little by little. The consistency you are looking for is not powdery or thick. The oatmeal should be moistened enough so you can handle it and apply it to the skin, but not so much it is sticky.

To use

This recipe needs to be made fresh each time you use it. Take handfuls of the mixture and massage into the skin. Use on the face, thighs and buttocks. Shower to remove.

Mint Body Scrub

Fresh mint and ground rice combine with soothing yogurt for a gentle exfoliating mask.

Ingredients

1 small container live natural yogurt
2 sprigs fresh peppermint, or 2 tsp (10 ml) dried
1 sprig fresh spearmint, or 2 tsp (10 ml) dried
1 cup (240 ml) ground rice

To make

Mix the yogurt and mints together and refrigerate for at least twenty four hours. The mint will infuse the yogurt. Stir the rice into the yogurt mixture. Do not grind the rice too finely and try to use brown rice, as the extra bran is good for the skin.

To use

This preparation needs to be made fresh each time you use it. The yogurt must be live, as the natural "friendly" bacteria liven up the skin and soothe to counteract the rough, exfoliating rice. This is a good all over exfoliator.

Ginger Skin Energizer

Ginger's warming effects can be felt in the tingle that is present after using this wonderful dead skin remover.

Ingredients

1 gingerroot, about 4 in (10 cm)
2 tbsp (30 ml) baking soda
2 tbsp (30 ml) kaolin

To make

Peel the gingerroot, and grate finely. Add the baking soda and the kaolin and mix everything together.

To use

This recipe needs to be made fresh each time you use it in order to make the most of the invigorating fresh enzymes from the ginger. This exfoliator is best used in the bath on sluggish areas, and it is warming—great on cold days. You may use it on the face, but make sure the ginger is puréed rather than grated or it may be too harsh for delicate facial skin.

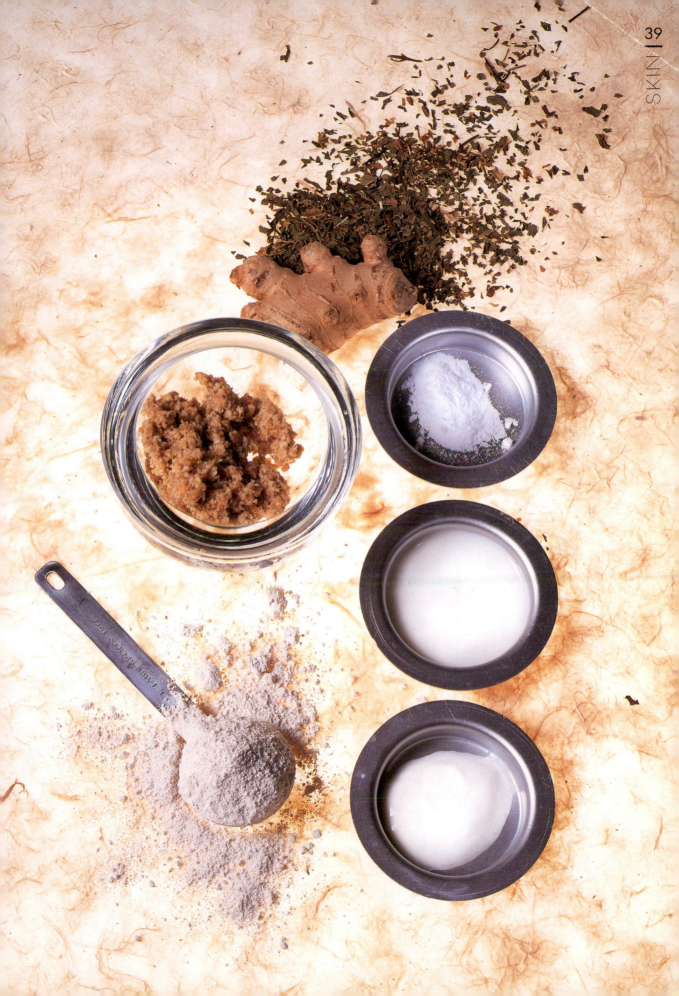

SKIN COMPLAINTS

Blemishes and skin complaints are often a problem for young people, and poor diet and lack of exercise can play a negative role. Too much washing can strip skin of its natural sebum (oil). This can cause overproduction of oil as a reaction, leading to blackheads. Skin looks healthy if the inside of the body is healthy, so monitoring your diet and even watching stress levels is very important to maintain healthy skin. For women, skin quality can vary with the menstrual cycle. Certain foods can help to balance hormones in this case (see the diet section).

improving skin quality

Sage and Comfrey Gel

Aloe vera base combined with an infusion of soothing sage and antiseptic comfrey (knitbone).

Ingredients

4 tbsp (60 ml) aloe vera gel

2 tbsp (30 ml) sage (preferably fresh)

2 tbsp (30 ml) comfrey

1 drop tea tree essential oil (optional)

To make

Very simple! Make sure the gel is cold so it doesn't thin too much when you start to work with it. Make a strong infusion with the herbs by immersing them in just enough hot water to cover them and leaving for at least two hours. Remove the herbs from the infusion and start to blend the liquid with the gel. You do not want the gel to become too thin, so you may not need all the infusion.

To use

Either apply to the whole face in a thin film and allow to dry before using makeup (use instead of a moisturizer) or use it directly on individual blemishes, adding a drop of tea tree essential oil in this case.

Tea Tree Face Mask

Cooling peppermint in a green clay base draws out dirt and impurities.

Ingredients

2 tbsp (30 ml) green clay
   (see page 16)

2 sprigs peppermint, or
   2 tsp (10 ml) dried

2 drops tea tree essential oil

To make

This preparation needs to be made fresh every time you wish to use it, because the clay will only remain fluid enough to handle while it is warm. Cover the peppermint leaves with hot water and leave to infuse for a few minutes. Remove the leaves and add the warm infusion to the clay and mix vigorously. The mixture should form a paste—if it is too solid add more hot water. Add the tea tree oil and mix in thoroughly.

To use

Apply to the skin warm, before the clay becomes crusty. Remove when thoroughly dry; the skin will be tightened and cleansed. Moisturize afterward.

Fresh Lemon Mask

Made from lemons and lemon balm herbal tincture, this is an astringent for open pores and oily skin.

Ingredients

1 lemon

1 egg white

1 tbsp (15 ml) lemon balm tincture

To make

Finely grate the lemon peel and squeeze the juice. Beat the egg white until foamy, just to separate and lighten it a little. Add the juice of the lemon and some grated rind. Add the tincture to create a light brown liquid —do not add too much or the mixture will be too runny.

To use

Egg white tightens the skin beautifully. It was widely used in Victorian times for this purpose as a base for makeup. Apply to the face and remove when the skin starts to feel tight. Do not remove with very hot water or the egg white will soften and solidify!

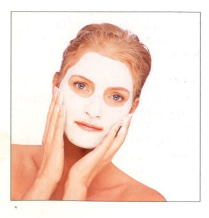

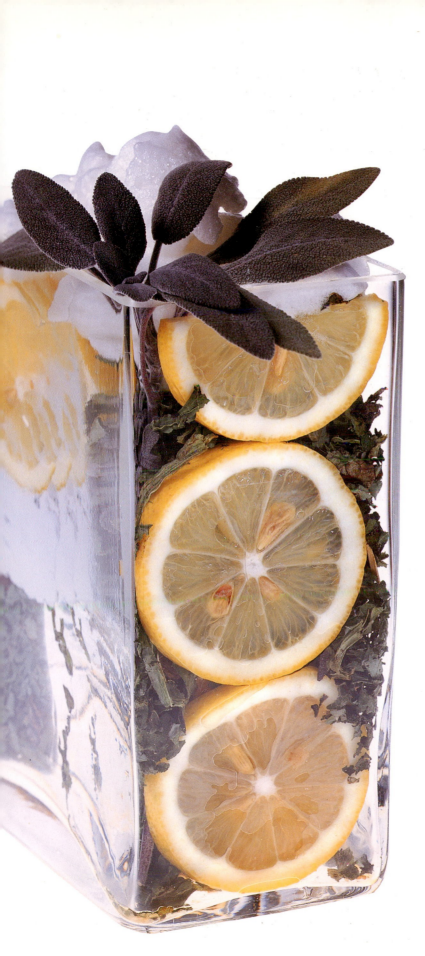

Evening Primrose Moisturizer

This recipe contains special fatty acids (GLA) and rose geranium oil, which balances hormones and can reduce acne.

Ingredients

2 tbsp (30 ml) base cream
2 drops vitamin E oil
1 evening primrose oil capsule (or more)
2 drops rose geranium essential oil

To make

Mix the cream, vitamin E and contents of the capsule together. You can buy evening primrose oil capsules from any health-food store (try to buy a small quantity, as they are expensive). You will need about 150–300 mg of GLA (evening primrose oil) in this cream. Extract the oil from the capsule by piercing the capsule with a pin and squirting out the contents. Add the rose geranium oil last and mix thoroughly.

To use

This cream is extremely rich. I suggest using it every day until the skin condition settles, then using every other day. You may also wish to take an evening primrose supplement at the same time.

SUN PROTECTION

The harmful rays of the sun can play havoc with your complexion and may lead to premature aging. These recipes will ensure an even tan, but they do not act as sunblocks or replace protective suntan creams. In order to create sun "block" of any kind chemicals such as octyl dimethyl PABA (UVB block) or titanium dioxide (UVA block) must be added to products. I suggest you buy sun care products from a reputable natural health outlet. To try and make them in your own home to the standard required for safety would be difficult and potentially hazardous.

sun creams

Safe Sun Tips

- Never stay out in exposed sun light between 12 noon and 3 PM on hot days.

- Take extra care to cover vulnerable areas such as the back of the neck and nose.

- Remember thin clothes do not always offer good enough protection against the sun.

- Use a waterproof sunblock, or reapply after swimming.

- Watch out for moles—these are the start locations for many types of skin cancer.

- Drink lots of water to prevent dehydration.

- Never expose a baby of under six months old to direct sunlight.

Lavender Sun Cream

Cocoa butter base combined with a soothing extract of lavender has a lovely fragrant aroma.

Ingredients

*Small block of cocoa butter
    (approximately ½ cup/120 ml)*

2 tbsp (30 ml) base lotion

2 drops lavender essential oil

To make

Heat the cocoa butter in a bowl over a pan of lightly simmering water and gradually add the base lotion. You are looking for a thick lotion consistency. Do not add all of the lotion if it is not needed, but remember the preparation will thicken when it cools. Add the lavender oil and mix thoroughly. Decant into a small screw top jar.

To use

Apply in generous quantities to any area exposed to the sun. Remember also to use a sunblock, especially if your lotion is quite oily, as it will attract the sun.

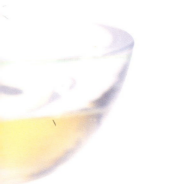

Lime and Peanut Tanning Oil

For those who do not burn easily or who have a good base tan, this oil is especially good for Asian or black skins. It induces a smooth, allover brown color. However, it does not provide sun protection.

Ingredients

4 tbsp (60 ml) sweet almond oil

4 tbsp (60 ml) peanut oil

2 drops lime essential oil

2 drops bergamot oil (optional)

To make

Mix all the ingredients together thoroughly in a screw-top bottle. The bergamot oil will really attract the sun, so only include this if you are not fair skinned and have a good base tan. Be sure to follow the safe sun tips also.

To use

Apply liberally. Not suitable for use on the face, as it is a bit heavy and the face often needs extra protection.

Lavender and Camomile After-sun Lotion

To soothe and calm angry, burning skin, this is easily absorbed and mild enough for the most sensitive skins.

Ingredients

2 drops lavender essential oil

2 drops camomile essential oil

4 tbsp (60 ml) base lotion

To make

Simply mix the oils thoroughly into the base lotion.

To use

Apply to the relevant area. It is also useful for heat rash and even insect bites.

Papaya Nourishing Salve

An intensely nourishing cream for moisture and tan preservation, it leaves the skin healthy and glowing due to the natural vitamin content and softening properties.

Ingredients

1 papaya

1 tbsp (15 ml) cocoa butter

To make

Remove the skin and seeds from the papaya and mash the soft fruit. Heat the cocoa butter either over hot water or directly on a spoon (watch out for heat transfer). Do not heat until runny, just softened. Mix the fruit and the cocoa butter, beating vigorously.

To use

Use immediately while the preparation is of the correct consistency. This recipe will not keep, so make enough for one application. (If you have leftover papaya, you can eat it. It really is delicious and in Africa it is thought to be a natural hormone regulator and contraceptive!) Apply to any dry peeling areas, leave only for a few moments before it becomes mushy, and shower to remove.

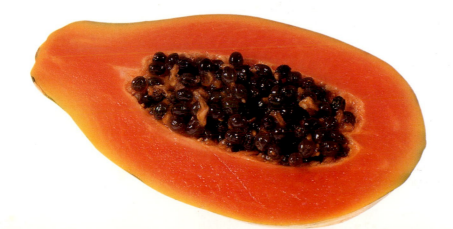

MATURE SKIN

As we get older the skin tightens and becomes less elastic. Essential oils that are good for increasing the elasticity of the skin are frankincense and orange (always dilute in a base oil). You may find your skin is drier as you mature, so using a rich vitamin E oil may be useful; for very dry skins try wheatgerm oil (these oils are also good for reducing stretch marks during pregnancy or weight fluctuation). Facial massage is another great way of reducing sagging and tightening the muscles.

treatments for older skin

Increasing muscle tone can reduce wrinkling. This needs to be done while the skin is still young as well as when it is mature. One way to do this successfully is through invigorating facial massage. Try the following step-by-step method for a self facial:

1) Start by gently stroking the face in an upward movement as if you are massaging a smile into place.

2) Smooth any "worry lines" around the forehead and eyebrows.

3) Gently pinch the eyebrows to release any pent up tension.

4) Lightly pat the face all over with the fingertips, like raindrops.

5) Gently pat the chin in an upward direction to encourage firming of the chin and neck muscles.

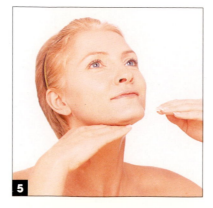

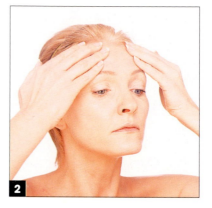

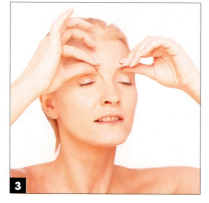

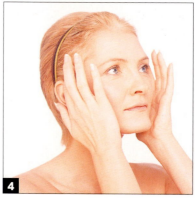

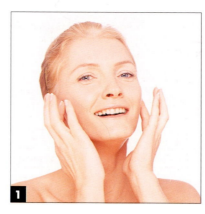

Grapefruit Puff

This is more of a dessert than a beauty treatment! Fresh grapefruit juice tightens and uplifts, while egg white nourishes and provides the skin with vital minerals.

Ingredients

1 egg white
1 tsp (5 ml) egg yolk
1 tbsp (15 ml) fresh grapefruit juice
1 drop vitamin E oil (optional)

To make

Beat the egg white until fluffy. Fold in the egg yolk and grapefruit juice, adding the oil if you want some extra richness and vitamin content. The mixture will thicken a little but try to keep in as much air as possible.

To use

Apply to the face and lie back while it works. Place cucumber slices over your eyes to cool and soothe while you wait. Do not try this mask in the bath or the steam will deflate the egg whites!

Traditional Face Cream

Here is a variation on an old fashioned, yet effective, cream for moisturizing the face.

Ingredients

2 tbsp (30 ml) rose water
2 tbsp (30 ml) almond oil
1 tbsp (15 ml) beeswax (optional)
2 tbsp (30 ml) aloe vera gel or juice

To make

Mix the rose water and almond oil thoroughly. You may find they have a tendency to separate, so you can either add some beeswax and heat for a more solid result or add less rose water until it is a thick, creamy consistency. Fold in the gel, using the amount needed to get the consistency you require.

To use

Use as a normal moisturizer, morning and evening, after cleansing and toning.

Body Powder

Delicate and luxurious, the body powder may be used after bathing to dust the skin and add a subtle fragrance.

Ingredients

1 cup (240 ml) dried rose petals
1 cup (240 ml) dried orange flowers
1 cup (240 ml) lavender flowers
1 cup (240 ml) orris root powder

To make

Make sure all the ingredients are thoroughly dry and remove any stalks or leaves. The orris root powder helps blend the other ingredients and slightly locks in the fragrance. The ingredients need to be pulverized together, ideally in a blender, or in a mortar and pestle by hand. You can use the powder immediately, but it will be best if you seal it in a plastic bag and leave it in a dry place for a couple of weeks.

To use

Applied all over the body, it leaves a soft shimmer and fragrance.

VISIBLE VEINS

The appearance of veins can be improved and swelling reduced with these simple recipes. Varicose veins are the result of blood pressure in a particular vein becoming so great that a vein valve bursts. Unfortunately, once a vein is damaged this process cannot be reversed. However, if you follow the guidelines below you can help to avoid further damage and care for already damaged veins.

caring for your legs

- Spend at least ten minutes a day with your legs raised as high as you can get them, longer if you spend a lot of time on your feet.

- Do not put a lot of pressure on an existing varicose vein, as you risk causing further damage. Avoid overexercising it and do not wear support hosiery, which restricts the blood flow.

- Seek medical advice if you have a varicose vein forming or a vein causing you a lot of pain.

- Do not underexercise, sluggishness can also make this condition worse.

Soothing Camomile Rinse

This is good used in a bath and especially suitable for the legs. It reduces swelling and discomfort at the end of a long day. The camomile smells wonderful.

Ingredients

3–4 tbsp (45–60 ml) dried camomile flowers

3–4 tbsp (45–60 ml) dried calendula flowers

3–4 tbsp (45–60 ml) dried arnica flowers (if you can get them)

To make

Make a giant "tea bag" by tying the herbs in cheesecloth. Put this bag under the running water of your bath and allow the infusion to seep into the bath water.

To use

Bathe in the water infused. For an extra boost rub the "tea bag" over your legs and buttocks.

Geranium and Clay Rejuvenator

Geraniums have natural draining properties, and this improves the appearance of small visible red capillaries under the skin. It is mixed with absorbent kaolin.

Ingredients

6 tbsp (90 ml) fresh geranium flowers or 2 drops geranium essential oil

1 cup (240 ml) kaolin

2 tbsp (30 ml) coarse ground rice

To make

Break up the geranium flowers by hand; randomly breaking splits the cell walls of the flowers, releasing all the natural goodness, and cutting with scissors will not have the same effect. Mix the flowers with the kaolin. If you are using essential oil instead make sure you mix it in thoroughly so it does not congeal with small clumps of the clay. Add the rice and mix again well.

To use

Rub into the legs and affected areas, and leave for at least ten minutes. If you prefer, you can mix the preparation with water to make a thick paste that will dry a few minutes after application.

CELLULITE

Cellulite may be alleviated if the correct changes to diet and lifestyle are made. Basically caused by a buildup of toxins under the fatty layers of the skin, the condition can be improved by avoiding tea, coffee, cigarettes and alcohol. Also, persistent cellulite can be shifted with a detoxification program involving drinking plenty of water and applying some good, homemade anticellulite preparations, along with regular exfoliating to boost circulation (use a loofah or other natural skin brush). Include more fruit and vegetables in your diet. Two-thirds of our diet is often "empty calories": sugars, white flour and processed food. They have little nutritional value, but cause weight gain, as they are stored as fat rather than moving through the digestive system or being burned as energy. For this reason, you do not have to be overweight to have cellulite.

preventive treatments

Juniper and Horsetail Treatment
Crushed juniper berries mixed with a strong infusion of cleansing horsetail herb are excellent for an occasional anticellulite boost.

Ingredients

6 tbsp (90 ml) juniper berries
3 tbsp (45 ml) horsetail herb

To make

Try to get hold of fresh juniper berries. They will be purple in color and juicy when fresh—they blacken and dry up with age. Crush the juniper berries with the back of a spoon in the bowl you are using to make the preparation in order to preserve all the juices. Mix the crushed berries with the horsetail herb and cover with just enough boiling water to submerge all the herbs. Leave to infuse until the water is cool.

To use

You can add the whole concoction to your bathwater and use the berries on a sponge to massage into your thighs.

Alternatively, remove the berries and herb, mix the liquid with some base cream and use as a lotion on cellulite areas after bathing.

Cellulite Oil

Use this after a hot bath when the skin is soft. It may be massaged into the affected areas and contains lymphatic drainers. Used around the chest and upper arms it helps to remove toxins from the body before they are stored. It contains rosemary to improve circulation, fennel and juniper to detoxify.

Ingredients

4 tbsp (60 ml) sweet almond oil
2 drops rosemary essential oil
2 drops fennel essential oil
2 drops juniper essential oil

To make

Put all ingredients in a screw-top bottle and shake vigorously to mix.

To use

Apply to the affected areas, massaging in deeply.

Strawberry and Ginger Reviver

This wakes up sluggish thighs and buttocks with a combination of active enzymes and warming stimulation.

Ingredients

1 gingerroot, about 4 in (10 cm)
2 tbsp (30 ml) kaolin
7 or 8 large strawberries

To make

Put all ingredients into a blender and whiz for a minute or so, until all the ginger is puréed with the other ingredients. This recipe is quick and easy, but you do need a blender, as the ginger will be too tough to work with by hand and the clay needs to expand and become sticky. If the mix seems a bit runny, you can add more clay to thicken.

To use

This recipe is so simple yet incredibly effective, and it also smells wonderful. Apply the fresh mixture onto sluggish skin and leave to dry for a few minutes.

HAIR

Hair can transform the way you look. However, popular products can damage the hair shaft and dry or strip the hair. Modern products that contain B vitamins help to counteract this process, although it makes more sense to make sure your diet includes enough vitamin B and work from the inside out. Preservatives in hair products can irritate the scalp and may even lead to dandruff. Overuse of products such as gel and mousse on the hair can cause buildup and irritate the scalp. A good quality shampoo, which is freshly made, along with the occasional deep conditioning treatment, is all your hair really needs.

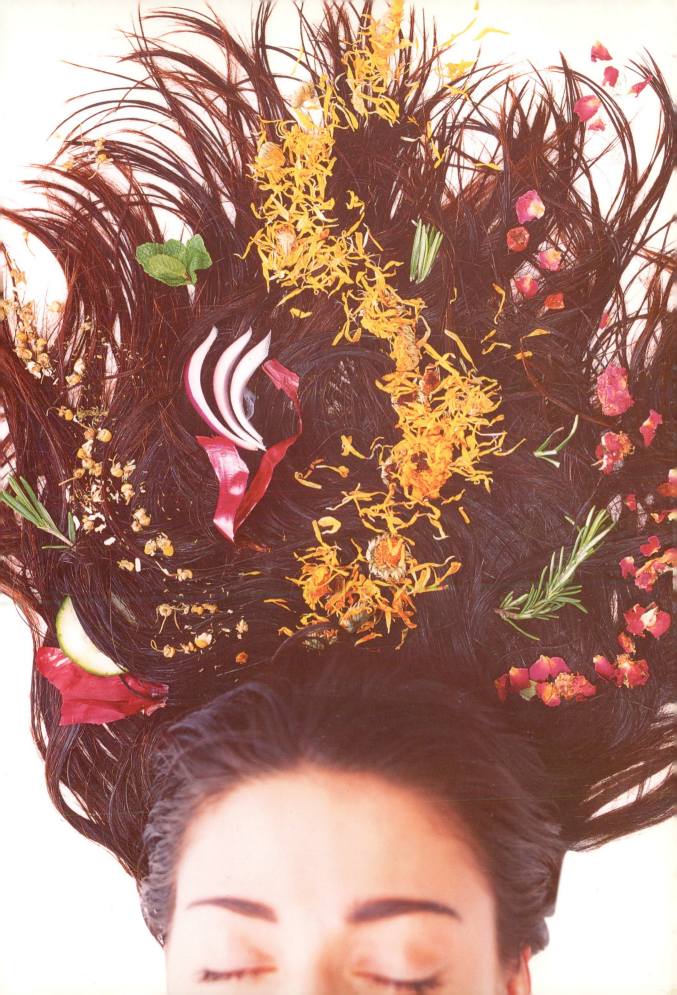

CLEANSING

Most of the shampoo recipes in this section use a shampoo base that has been purchased and is not homemade. You can make your own shampoo base but it is a complicated and messy job, probably not worth the effort, because a small error in quantity will affect the consistency of the end result significantly and can mean much waste of time and ingredients. It is fairly easy to buy organic base shampoos and I would recommend this. Certainly do not buy anything fragranced or containing additives. Some of the shampoo recipes do not contain this base shampoo and are formulated from herbal infusions. These are most suitable for people with sensitive skin or hair.

shampoos

Coconut and Orange Solid Shampoo

For dry hair, this shampoo has a coconut oil solid base that is extremely nourishing. When left in the hair for five minutes it cleanses and conditions.

Ingredients

2 tbsp (30 ml) coconut oil

3 drops orange essential oil

1 drop bois de rose oil

To make

Heat the coconut oil in a bowl over hot water. Off the heat, add the essential oils and blend thoroughly. Pour into a screw-top jar and leave to harden.

To use

Apply in small quantities combing from the roots through the hair. Leave on for at least five minutes. Rinse off. You may find it difficult to remove all traces of the oil. You can leave it in the hair, creating soft and shiny hair, or thoroughly rinse with a plain base shampoo that lathers.

Combination Shampoo and Conditioner

Convenient and easy, this is good for traveling.

Ingredients

4 tbsp (60 ml) shampoo base

3–4 tbsp (45–60 ml) calendula petals

2 drops lavender essential oil

To make

Put the shampoo base and flowers into a large jar. Mix in the essential oil thoroughly and seal. Leave at room temperature to infuse for at least a week and up to two months. The calendula flowers infuse their cleansing and conditioning properties into the base. After infusing, remove the flowers from the shampoo and put into a dispenser bottle.

To use

Shampoo as usual. Your hair will also be lightly conditioned.

Geranium and Petitgrain Light Shampoo

An effective yet gentle cleanser, petitgrain is good for sensitive scalps and oily hair.

Ingredients

4 tbsp (60 ml) base shampoo

2 drops petitgrain essential oil

2 drops geranium essential oil

To make

Just mix all ingredients thoroughly and put into a dispenser bottle.

To use

Shampoo. You will only need to apply and rinse once.

shampoos

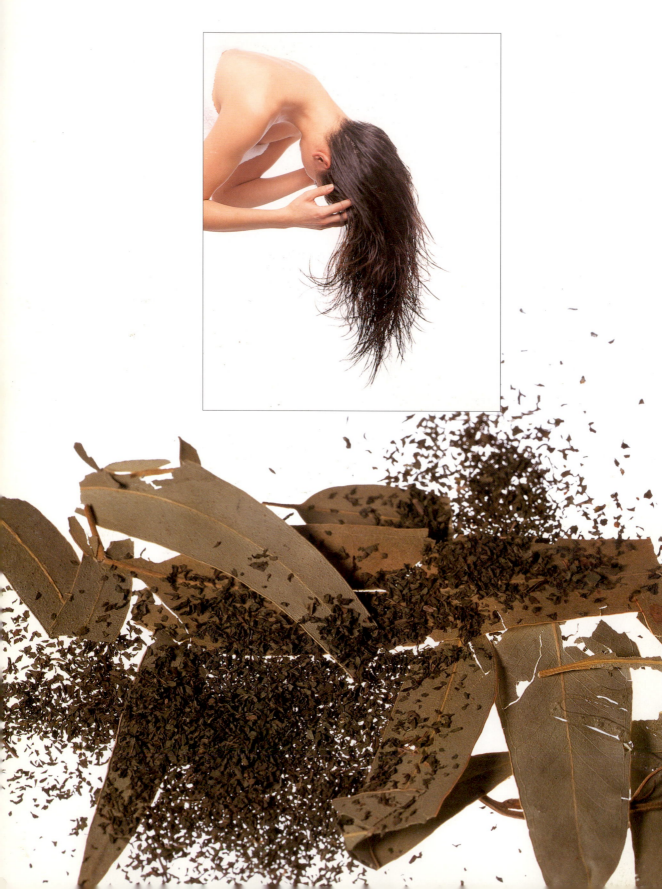

Detoxifying Shampoo

For occasional use only, this infusion of peppermint, eucalyptus leaves and fresh strawberries stimulates enzyme action.

Ingredients

4 or 5 strawberries
2 tbsp (30 ml) shampoo base
2 tbsp (30 ml) peppermint leaves
2 tbsp (30 ml) eucalyptus leaves

To make

Mash the strawberries, either by hand or in a blender, and mix with the shampoo base. If the mixture looks very runny do not add all the strawberries. Leave overnight in the refrigerator. Meanwhile, infuse the peppermint and eucalyptus in a small amount of very hot water (see page 15). When the water has cooled, strain and blend with the strawberry base, a little at a time, until it forms a thin paste.

To use

Shampoo as usual. It will not lather too much, but this is fine. Rinse hair well to remove the strawberry seeds.

CONDITIONING

Careful conditioning will prevent your hair from becoming tangled and can also improve dry or damaged hair. Brushing the hair carefully and regularly can also benefit its condition. Brushing separates the hair, leaving it looking fuller, and also cleanses it by dislodging tangles and dirt. You don't really need to condition your hair every time you wash it. If you have oily hair, try every other time. However, if you swim often, do condition regularly, as chlorine dries out hair.

recipes for conditioners

Herbal Conditioner

This is a light conditioner, so it's great for those with oily hair. Lemongrass is cleansing and mildly astringent. Ginseng helps bring life and vitality to the hair.

Ingredients

5 drops ginseng tincture
1 tbsp (15 ml) lemongrass
4 tbsp (60 ml) grapeseed oil

To make

The ginseng tincture is an alcohol-based herbal extract. Korean ginseng is the best, but often the most expensive. Store the lemongrass in the oil for at least two weeks, longer if you can be patient (maximum two months). The fragrance and properties of the lemongrass are imported to the oil in this way. Strain the oil and mix in the tincture shaking vigorously to blend. Each time you use this conditioner, shake the bottle to make sure the alcohol in the ginseng tincture is well dispersed.

To use

Apply as a normal conditioner but before shampooing. Allow to remain on the hair for at least five minutes. A steamy bath or hot shower is a good place to apply this treatment, as the steam helps the conditioning process. Shampoo and rinse.

Nettle and Onion Rinse

It sounds a little peculiar, but Native Americans have used onion for centuries to add shine to the hair. The nettles have a fresh smell to counteract that of the onions.

Ingredients

1 small onion
3 tbsp (45 ml) dried nettle leaves

To make

Cut the onion into quarters; try not to separate it any more than this. Crush the nettles (they need to be dried; fresh nettles become too soggy in the infusion). Put all ingredients in a large bowl and cover with really hot water. Allow to infuse (see page 15) for half an hour (no longer or it will be mushy and you will have steamed onions!) Strain the liquid and refrigerate.

To use

Best used fresh after half an hour cooling in the refrigerator. When cold this tonic is even more invigorating; it gets everything going, boosting circulation. Wash your hair as usual and use this preparation before the final rinse.

Jojoba and Vanilla Treatment

An excellent overnight application for all hair types, especially dry hair, it removes grime and helps to seal split ends.

Ingredients

2 tbsp (30 ml) jojoba oil
2 tsp (10 ml) apricot kernel oil
1 vanilla pod

To make

Mix the oils together in a screw-top jar. Place the vanilla pod in the oil and leave to infuse for at least three days before using. Do not refrigerate, as this will solidify the jojoba oil, which is actually a liquid wax, and it will slow the infusion process.

To use

Apply to dry hair and leave for at least an hour but preferably overnight (wrap your hair in an old scarf or towel to avoid staining your pillow case). If you have long hair, tie it up to avoid drying out. Comb the conditioner through to the ends of the hair. If you have very dry, curly hair, now is a chance to comb it through thoroughly. Rinse off in the normal way, or you may wish to shampoo for squeaky clean hair.

NATURAL COLOR

Natural hair color enhancers are gentle and do not strip the hair. They work on the shine and color you have, rather than removing and replacing existing color with harsh chemicals. Henna can also be used as a natural colorant; this will change the color for a longer time. Neutral henna does not color hair, it just enhances shine. Henna can cover small amounts of gray hair.

colors and shiners

Rosemary Infusion

For dark hair, this enhances natural color and it highlights red tones.

Ingredients

2 tbsp (30 ml) rosemary leaves

1 tbsp (15 ml) thyme leaves

To make

Cover the herbs with very hot (not boiling) water, leave to infuse for at least two hours (see page 15). Strain. Try to use fresh herbs as these have more fresh enzyme action. The stronger the infusion the more effect it will have.

To use

Apply the infusion to the hair after shampooing, before your final rinse. Leave it on the hair as long as possible. Steam from a hot bath will help the process. You can comb the infusion through the hair and leave on overnight (wrap your hair in a scarf so it doesn't stain your pillow). It will leave a lovely herbal fragrance on your hair.

Yucca Hair Mask

A real miracle worker, yucca brings a rich shine to lackluster hair.

Ingredients

2–3 tbsp (30–45 ml) yucca root

2–3 tbsp (30–45 ml) birch leaves

2–3 tbsp (30–45 ml) alder herb

2 tbsp (30 ml) vodka

To make

Cover the herbs with a small amount of very hot (not boiling) water and leave to infuse for at least thirty minutes. Strain and add the vodka after the liquid has cooled (or the preserving alcohol will evaporate).

To use

The yucca will make the tonic a pale brown color, so do not worry about this. You can comb the tonic into your hair and leave it overnight or wash out immediately. If you have dry hair, condition it well, as the alcohol content in this recipe is quite high and it may dry your hair a little.

Camomile Infusion

Make in exactly the same way as the rosemary infusion, but use 4 tbsp (60 ml) camomile instead. Camomile enhances the blond in light hair. Adding some honey to the final rinse can condition the hair even more. Use runny honey and dilute it in hot water so it doesn't become too sticky.

Red Onion Rinse

This brings out the color of auburn hair—with dramatic results.

Ingredients

1 small red onion

2 tbsp (30 ml) malt vinegar

To make

Chop the onion and leave it to infuse in the vinegar topped up with warm water to cover for twenty four hours. Do not use hot water or the onion will start to cook. Strain after this time.

To use

Use as a rinse after washing your hair. You may wish to comb it into your hair and leave for a period of time. The fragrance is not very pleasant, so follow with a fresh shampoo or conditioner.

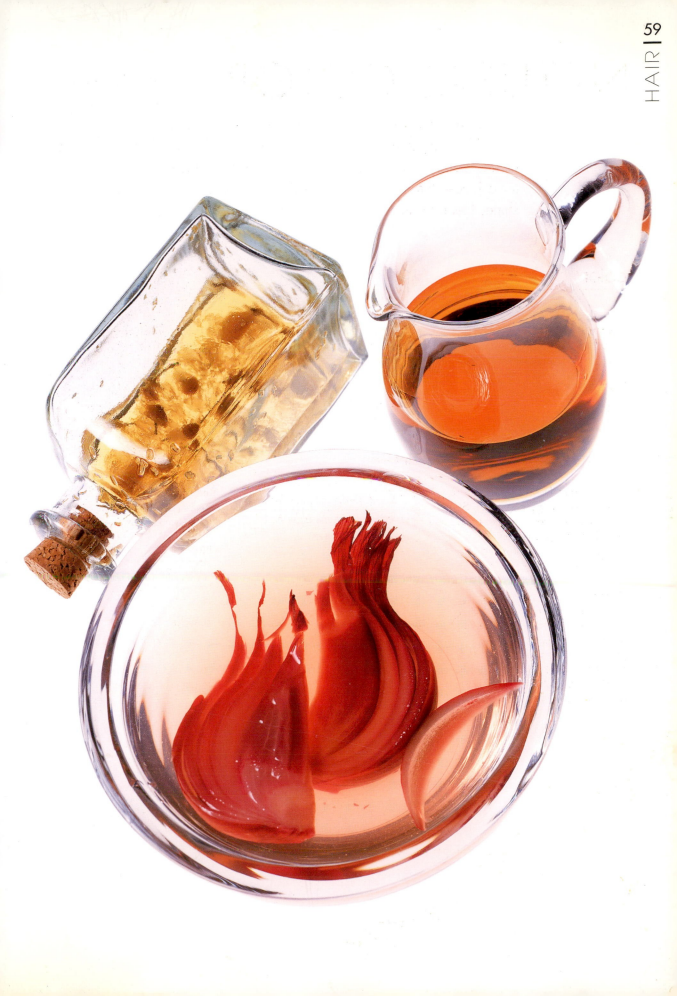

DANDRUFF

Dandruff is often a sign that the body is run down, or that vital vitamins or minerals are lacking from the diet. Often this is vitamin E. Unfortunately, many of the dandruff treatments you can buy irritate the scalp further, when gentle treatment is needed. Rinsing with cold water when you wash your hair is said to help prevent dandruff by keeping the scalp skin healthy.

treatments for scalp conditions

Carrot and Honey Hair Mask

Carotene is moisturizing and nourishing. It improves the condition of the scalp and makes hair shiny.

Ingredients

2 carrots

1 tbsp (15 ml) thick honey

2 tbsp (30 ml) oatmeal

1 tsp (5 ml) sweet almond oil (optional)

To make

Grate the carrot skins (not the inside part of the carrot, as this is too mushy). Mix grated carrot and other ingredients together to form a thick paste. If the consistency is too thick, add a little sweet almond oil, but take care to blend thoroughly.

To use

This mask is very sticky, so you will need to shampoo thoroughly after using it. Apply to the hair and leave for a few minutes, then wash out. It is best on short hair but can get a bit messy on long hair.

Yogurt and Myrrh Conditioner

Antifungal and antibacterial, this conditioner is cooling for itchy, red scalps.

Ingredients

Half a cucumber

1 small container live natural yogurt

1 tsp (5 ml) myrrh tincture

To make

If you have a blender, whiz everything together. If not, grate the cucumber and mix with the other ingredients. Refrigerate to cool for half an hour. Myrrh is a strong antifungal agent.

To use

Apply to the head quickly to make the most of the fresh ingredients and enzymes. Use cool, straight from the refrigerator, applying the mixture to the head and scalp more than the hair. Leave for a few minutes and rinse to remove. The cucumber is wonderfully soothing and gives this recipe a cool, fresh scent.

Eucalyptus and Kaolin Deep Cleaning Shampoo

The scalp and hair right down to the roots are deeply cleansed. This preparation invigorates and removes dead skin, reaching the parts other cleansers cannot!

Ingredients

3 tbsp (45 ml) kaolin

2 tsp (10 ml) ground rice (you can buy it ground, or grind it yourself in a small coffee grinder)

3 drops eucalyptus essential oil

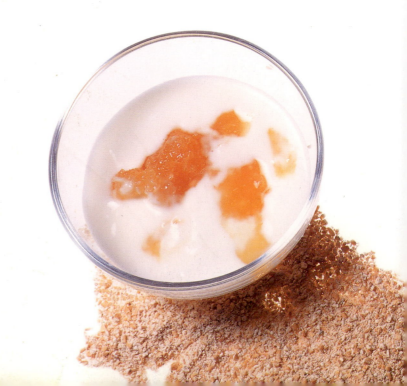

To make

Mix the kaolin and rice thoroughly.
Do not grind the rice too finely.
Add the essential oil and blend
with your fingers to make sure it is
thoroughly dispersed. You will have
a dry mixture the consistency of
breadcrumbs. This will keep for a
long time, best in a refrigerator.

To use

Take a small amount of the
mixture and add water to make
into a paste, then apply the
paste to the roots of the hair
and scalp, this is easiest on short
hair. Leave for at least ten minutes
and rinse. The eucalyptus will
leave your head tingly and your hair
will be shiny.

Camomile and Calendula Rinse

A stronger preparation for psoriasis
or very itchy scalps. The wheat germ
oil soothes and provides a valuable
source of vitamin E.

Ingredients

2 tbsp (30 ml) camomile flowers

2 tbsp (30 ml) shampoo base

1 tsp (5 ml) calendula tincture

1 tsp (5 ml) wheat germ oil

To make

Leave the camomile flowers to infuse
(see page 15) in the shampoo base
at least overnight, then remove. Add
the tincture to the base and then
gradually, the oil. You may not need
all the oil: the consistency should be
that of an oily shampoo.

To use

Shampoo as usual, but really
massage into the roots thoroughly. If
the mixture is very oily, shampoo the
hair with some plain base shampoo
afterwards.

SUN PROTECTION

Hair also needs protection from the sun, especially dry or brittle hair. Leaving some coconut oil in the hair when outside in the sunshine can help to protect it, especially at the ends, where hair tends to split and dry out. If you are swimming in the sea or a pool remember that salt and chlorine also have a drying effect on the hair, so you will need to use extra moisturizing conditioners.

hair in the sun treatments

Protective Hair Tonic

This prevents excess drying of the hair shaft and seals and strengthens the hair.

Ingredients

1 tbsp (15 ml) alder herb
1 tbsp (15 ml) dried nettle leaves
1 tbsp (15 ml) dried rosemary leaves
1 tbsp (15 ml) vodka

To make

Cover the herbs with very hot water and leave to infuse (see page 15) for at least two hours. Strain the herbs and cool the liquid. Add the vodka.

To use

Comb into the hair before swimming or sunbathing. You can leave in the hair for as long as you like; it does make hair shiny and soft.

DRY SCALP

A dry and itchy scalp is not only uncomfortable, it may also look unsightly. Many of the shampoos on the market for this problem are very strong and may irritate sensitive skin further. In an extreme case your doctor may prescribe steroids, which will help shortterm, but remember your body quickly becomes tolerant to them and you may find yourself in the position of needing more to achieve the same effect. I suggest treating a sensitive scalp with very gentle shampoos and conditioners; especially do not over treat it by washing your hair too often.

hair strengtheners

HAIR GROWTH

Although little can be done to actually make the hair grow, strengthening it and stimulating the hair shaft can be helpful.

Rosemary and Beer Tonic

These two ingredients are reputed to stimulate the hair shaft and promote growth.

Ingredients

2 drops rosemary essential oil
1 bottle strong ale or stout
1 drop tangerine essential oil (optional)

To make

Mix the rosemary oil into the ale and leave for at least twenty four hours. The beer itself contains alcohol, which is a natural preservative, so this recipe is very simple. If you wish to enhance the fragrance, add a drop of tangerine essential oil (not orange this could color the hair).

To use

Use before the final rinse after washing your hair. Beer is a traditional rinse for shiny hair, especially for brunettes.

SCALP PROBLEMS

Natural remedies can help cure scalp problems.

Peppermint and Tea Tree Shampoo

Simple yet effective for really dry problem scalps.

Ingredients

2 drops peppermint essential oil
2 drops tea tree essential oil
4 tbsp (60 ml) shampoo base

To make

Mix the oils thoroughly with the base.

To use

Shampoo as usual, leaving the lather in the hair for a few minutes before rinsing.

HANDS &

One of the most noticeable parts of the body, in addition to the face, are the hands. In any beauty regime, it is important to take care of the hands and nails. They are the most exposed area of the body, and are likely to be immersed in water and detergents more than any other body part. However, along with the feet, they have the most dense skin thickness. Dryness is often a problem, compounded by heating, air conditioning and exposure to the elements. The nails are actually living horny skin and can absorb moisturizer, although to a lesser extent than normal skin. Weak nails may also be strengthened by including more minerals in the diet or taking supplements.

NAILS

manicure

1) Wash hands with a gentle formula soap.

2) Immerse clean hands in bowl of warm water containing one drop of camomile essential oil and leave to soak for five minutes.

3) Dry hands, rub cuticle remover into nail bases and remove cuticles with an orange stick (see red elm cuticle softener recipe).

4) Moisturize hands, especially the cuticle area.

5) Apply nail polish if desired; use a base coat to avoid staining.

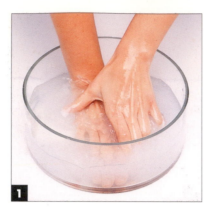

1

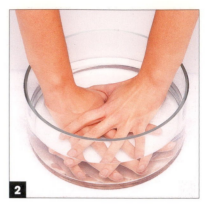

2

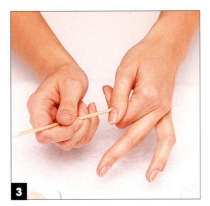

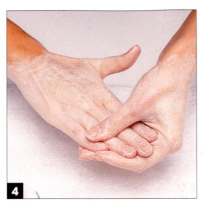

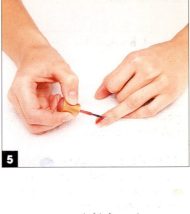

Nail Reviver

Cleansing lemon and nourishing sweet almond oil in a base of softening beeswax make a revitalizing treatment.

Ingredients

2 tsp (10 ml) beeswax
2 drops lemon essential oil
2 tbsp (30 ml) sweet almond oil

To make

Heat the beeswax in a small bowl over simmering water. When the beeswax is runny, mix in the lemon oil thoroughly, then add the almond oil little by little; you may not need it all. As the beeswax hardens you will get a sense of the final consistency; it should be solid but pliable. Transfer the mixture into a small jar.

To use

Apply to the fingertips and nails regularly, especially in cold weather. Massage into the skin thoroughly. If nails are weak, keeping them short until they strengthen will help.

Olive Oil Conditioner for Hands

The method employed for applying this recipe is a bit unusual, but wearing plastic gloves is very effective.

Ingredients

2 tbsp (30 ml) olive oil
2 drops orange essential oil
1 drop frankincense essential oil

To make

Mix all the oils together in a bottle. Orange and frankincense are very nourishing.

To use

This is especially good as an overnight treatment for very dry hands. The best way to apply it is to thoroughly immerse the hands in the oil and then get somebody to help you put on thin plastic gloves. Sleep with the treatment (and the gloves!) on. This gives very dry hands the chance to really heal. It is especially good for eczema on the hands. In the morning, rinse thoroughly and massage excess oil into the hands. The better the quality of olive oil, the more delicate the fragrance of the conditioner, so ideally use extra virgin, organic olive oil.

Red Elm Cuticle Softener

A red elm infusion with a beeswax base softens and removes hard skin.

Ingredients

2 tbsp (30 ml) red elm herb
1 tbsp (15 ml) jojoba oil
1 tbsp (15 ml) beeswax

To make

The quantities here are fairly small, but since this recipe is one that will keep longer than most, you can make up a slightly larger batch if you prefer. Put the herb in the jojoba oil and leave in a warm place to infuse for two weeks, but not much longer, as this is a strong herb and it will be too concentrated if left too long. Strain the herb from the oil and heat the oil slightly (it is a liquid wax and if overheated, it will not solidify when cooled). Add the beeswax and heat until melted, stirring. Transfer to a small jar and refrigerate to set.

To use

Rub the softener into the cuticles. To remove cuticles, take an orange stick and gently ease the softened skin of the cuticle off, leaving the nails smooth and shiny. This will encourage healthy new nail growth.

Apricot Kernel Rough Skin Remover

Made from apricot kernels, this fragrant scrub is gentle and effective.

Ingredients

2 tbsp (30 ml) apricot kernels
2 tbsp (30 ml) rice bran
1 tsp (5 ml) apricot kernel oil

To make

Whiz the apricot kernels in a blender until ground finely. Mix with the rice bran. Mix in enough oil to just form a paste. It should be a thick non-runny consistency.

To use

Take a small amount in the palm of damp, clean hands. Rub into the skin and rinse. The bran softens and exfoliates the skin, while the oil provides nourishing properties. It can also be used on the feet; just use less bran and more apricot kernels.

FEET

An often neglected part of the body, feet are abused by bad shoe design and the changes in temperature that can cause chilblains. Regular care can ensure soft, well-pedicured feet. Deodorizing feet can be a problem, especially in summer months when athletic shoes and synthetic materials can increase the problem. Commercial products on sale for deodorizing the feet can block the skin's pores and simply aggravate the problem, although deodorized innersoles for shoes may be helpful. Corns and calluses may develop on the feet as a result of poorly fitting shoes in childhood, as well as from stiletto heels and excessively pointed shoes later on. In severe cases you will need to visit a podiatrist to have these removed. However, looking after your feet now can prevent these problems in the future.

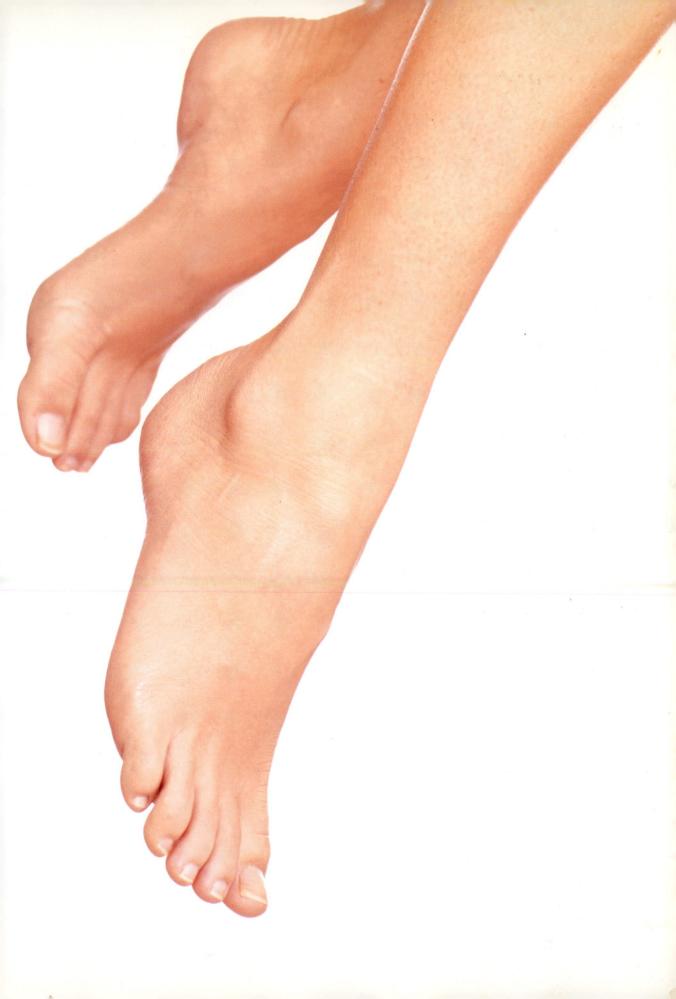

foot preparations

Kaolin and Mint Foot Powder

A rough, grainy talc with a clay base that absorbs moisture, this is good to rub onto the feet after bathing.

Ingredients

2 sprigs peppermint herb (dried)
¾ cup (180 ml) full white kaolin
2 drops peppermint essential oil
1 drop bois de rose essential oil

To make

You need to use dried peppermint, as fresh is too moist. Mix together the clay and essential oils until they resemble very fine breadcrumbs. Ideally use a blender, but make sure it is completely dry, or the moisture will clog the talc. You may also mix by hand, using the fingertips to "comb" the mixture. Add the peppermint last and mix well.

To use

Apply as usual. Be careful to keep the talc free of moisture when storing it, otherwise it will be unusable. Keep it in a sealed container, as clay will harden with the small amount of moisture from the air.

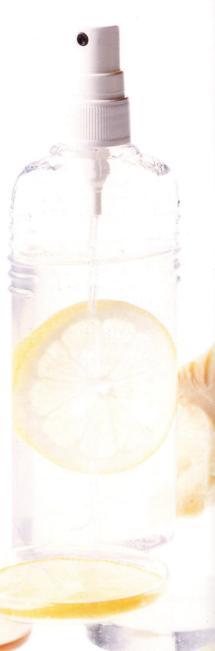

Tea Tree and Lemon Spray

Very simple but very effective, this spray is great in hot weather.

Ingredients

2 tsp (10 ml) fresh lemon juice
2 tbsp (30ml) vodka
2 tbsp (30ml) water
3 drops lemon essential oil
3 drops tea tree oil

To make

Use fresh lemon juice, as it is a natural preservative and will not oxidize. Put all the ingredients in a spray bottle and mix thoroughly.

To use

You will need to shake the bottle thoroughly each time you use this spray, to mix all the ingredients and disperse the essential oil. You can use it all over the feet to cool and deodorize. You can also use it on other body areas, but not the face, as the alcohol is drying.

Cocoa Butter and Calendula Rub

A thick cocoa butter base makes this rub intensely moisturizing.

Ingredients

2 tbsp (30 ml) of cocoa butter
2 tsp (10 ml) calendula tincture
2 tbsp (30 ml) calendula petals
1 tbsp (15 ml) camomile flowers

To make

Heat the cocoa butter in a small bowl over simmering water, then mix in the tincture. Add the flowers and mix again vigorously. You can use a blender, but the mixture will clog it if it is not runny enough. This recipe can be a bit messy, but it is worth experimenting with different varieties of cocoa butter until you get it right, as the results are worth the effort! You need softer cocoa butter than usual. If it comes in a hard block, try heating it then cooling, as this usually gives it a softer consistency.

To use

Use as a moisturizer and massage into the feet. The reflexology points are all on the soles of the feet, so massaging this area benefits the whole body.

foot treatments

Cucumber and Spearmint Foot Mask

This recipe is wonderfully soothing for tired feet after a long, hot day. This yoghurt based mask cools, relaxes and refreshes the feet.

Ingredients

1 small cucumber

2 drops spearmint essential oil

2 tbsp (30 ml) fresh spearmint herb

1 tbsp (15 ml) kaolin or green clay (see page 19)

6 tbsp (90 ml) natural yogurt

To make

Put all ingredients in a blender and whiz to mix thoroughly. The clay will help give the thick consistency needed. You can mix by hand, but it will take longer and the result will not amalgamate so well. This recipe has many variations. You can also use peppermint if spearmint is not available, but it is less refreshing; you will need less essential oil (1 drop) because it is generally stronger. Equally, you can use lemon balm and essential oil instead of mint for its deodorizing properties.

To use

Make up fresh each time you want to use it, to take advantage of the enzyme action of the cucumber. Use the ingredients straight from the refrigerator for a cooling foot mask. Cover feet in the mask, either over the bathtub or a bowl, to avoid unnecessary mess. Allow the mask to dry, and rinse with cool water to invigorate the skin.

Winter Warmer Foot Bath

Great for reviving cold feet in wintry weather, this treatment helps prevent chilblains.

Ingredients

1 tsp (5 ml) base dispersing oil or 1 tbsp (15 ml) whole milk
1 drop camomile essential oil
1 drop lavender essential oil
1 drop sandalwood essential oil
2 cups (480 ml) warm water

To make

The dispersing oil helps the essential oils mix into the water; otherwise you will have a few drops of oil on the surface of the water and nothing in the main foot bath. You can also substitute a tablespoon of whole milk, which has fat that acts as a dispersing agent. Mix all the ingredients in a large bowl.

To use

Immerse the feet and let the essential oils do their job. Rosemary is for circulation, sandalwood is soothing and lavender helps swelling.

EYES

Our eyes make more than 100,000 movements a day, so they deserve attention from time to time. We often neglect our eyes without realizing it, by exposing them to smoky environments or not removing eye makeup. It is important to allow the eye to function as it should and provide its own moisture. A healthy adult should rarely need eye drops. For the many people who suffer from conjunctivitis or hay fever, try bathing the eyes in an infusion of eyebright (one of several herbs of the *Euphrasia* genus traditionally used for eye ailments) or calendula. Never put essential oils (neat or dilute) in the eye area. Visual stress is a twentieth-century ailment caused by time spent looking at screens. Make sure conditions you work in are well lit, avoid straining to see something out of focus and have your eyes tested regularly.

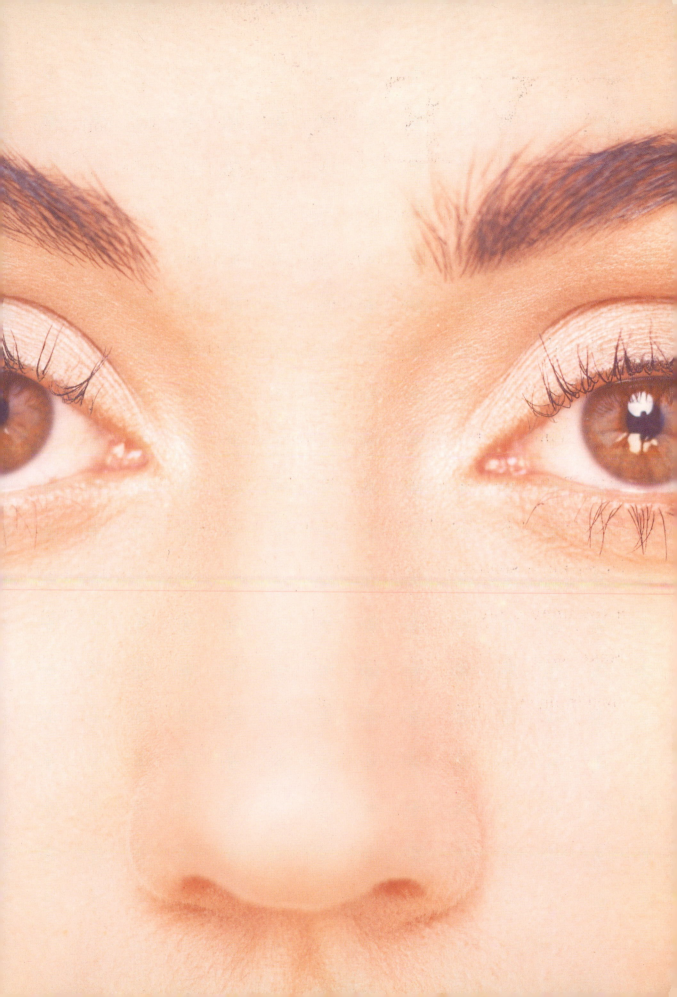

EYESTRAIN

Eyes often become tired and sore after a day spent in front of a computer screen or reading small print. Always make sure that you work in well-lit conditions, and if you suffer from eyestrain, have your eyes tested regularly. Tired eyes can become dry, and splashing your eyes with cold water will refresh them and stimulate the tiny eye capillaries. For an instant lift, relax with cucumber slices over the eye area.

relief for tired eyes

Eyebright Wash for Tired Eyes

A great pickup for tired eyes, this formula also helps counteract inflammation.

Ingredients

1 tsp (5 ml) eyebright herb
1 tsp (5 ml) chickweed herb
2 tbsp (30 ml) boiling water

To make

Cover the herbs with warm water and allow to infuse (see page 15) for at least ten minutes, but no more than twenty minutes or the chickweed becomes bitter. Strain and cool before use.

To use

Apply using an eye-bathing cup or on a medium-sized cotton pad. Change the cotton pad or eye bath contents each time you apply the solution, to avoid reinfection if you have conjunctivitis or any similar ailment. If you cool the infusion before use, this will have the effect of tightening the eye capillaries, thus resting and soothing them.

Cucumber Soother

Here is a quick and simple way to pep up tired eyes.

Ingredients

2 tea bags
1 small cucumber

To make

Immerse the tea bags in hot water, squeeze out excess moisture and leave to cool. Purée the cucumber in a blender or food processor, or grate very finely by hand. This recipe needs to be made just before using, as the enzyme action will not last.

To use

First close your eyes and lie back with the cool, wet teabags over them for a few minutes. Tea is mildly astringent and will cool and relax the eyes. Next, place the cucumber mixture over the eyes in the same way, avoiding contact with the actual eye itself. Again relax and let the cooling enzymes do their work. Rinse to remove and pat the eye area dry with a soft towel.

Green Tea Rinse

Green tea is extremely soothing and detoxifying. In Asia it is renowned for increasing life expectancy. It reduces swelling in the tiny, overworked eye muscles.

Ingredients

2 tbsp (30 ml) green tea leaves

3 drops vodka

To make

Cover the tea leaves with ½ cup (120 ml) boiling water and leave to infuse for at least twenty minutes. Boil the tea for fifteen minutes to evaporate some of the liquid, concentrating the infusion. Allow the mixture to cool thoroughly before adding and mixing in the vodka, otherwise this will also evaporate.

To use

Soak cotton balls in some of the rinse and dab onto the eye area. Alternatively, use an eye-bathing cup.

RECIPES FOR EYES

The cosmetics that we use on the face and especially around the eye area can sometimes do more harm than good and the delicate skin can easily become irritated by the application of eye makeup. To avoid problems set aside a day a week when you do not wear eye makeup, and always remove makeup at night by gently applying remover with cotton or soft tissue. Never rub the eye area.

eye treatments

Eyelash Thickener

This recipe will actually strengthen your eyelashes if used regularly, unlike ordinary mascara, which can weaken the hair shaft (to avoid this look for conditioning varieties).

Ingredients

1 tbsp (15 ml) beeswax
5 drops sweet almond oil
2 drops alder tincture
1 drop lemon essential oil

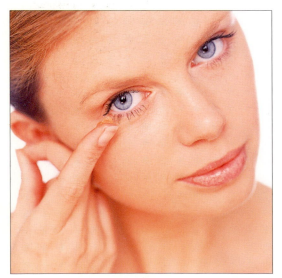

To make

Heat the beeswax in a small bowl over simmering water. When melted, add the almond oil and allow the mixture to cool slightly until it begins to solidify. Add the tincture and essential oil and mix well. Transfer to a small screw-top jar. The mixture will look like a thick gel.

To use

Apply a small amount with the fingertips. Do not apply too much or the eyelashes will stick together.

Natural Eye Makeup Remover

An extremely gentle cleanser, this will not irritate the eye and will help to rehydrate your skin.

Ingredients

4 tbsp (60 ml) jojoba oil
2 drops calendula tincture
1 drop mallow tincture
2 drops vodka

To make

Dispense the joboba oil in a small glass bottle. Add the tinctures and the vodka, a drop at a time. Working in amounts as small as drops can be tricky, so to avoid dropping them onto the side of the bottle, aim for the center of the oil. Mix ingredients by vigorously shaking the bottle.

To use

Apply in small quantities on cotton balls or a soft tissue.

Brewer's Yeast Supplement
Mix two teaspoons (10 ml) of
brewer's yeast supplement with
water and take internally on a daily
basis. This is reputed to remove
shadows from under the eyes.
Do not take if you have yeast
intolerance problems, and seek
advice from a qualified nutrition
expert if you are unsure about
taking any supplement.

MOUTH

Oral hygiene is an important part of grooming, often neglected. More than just cleaning our teeth, oral hygiene involves everything from maintaining fresh breath to silky, smooth lips. Smoking and alcohol consumption can all take their toll on oral hygiene. By brushing to prevent tooth decay and plaque buildup and making regular visits to the dentist, we can all avoid fillings and even tooth removal. It is important to use a good quality toothpaste that contains fluoride. Check whether you may also have fluoride added to your water supply. Too much fluoride in the system can be toxic and have an adverse effect. When cleaning your teeth, brush gently to avoid damage to the gums, but also thoroughly cover every area. Plenty of green leafy vegetables (B vitamins) will help ensure healthy gums.

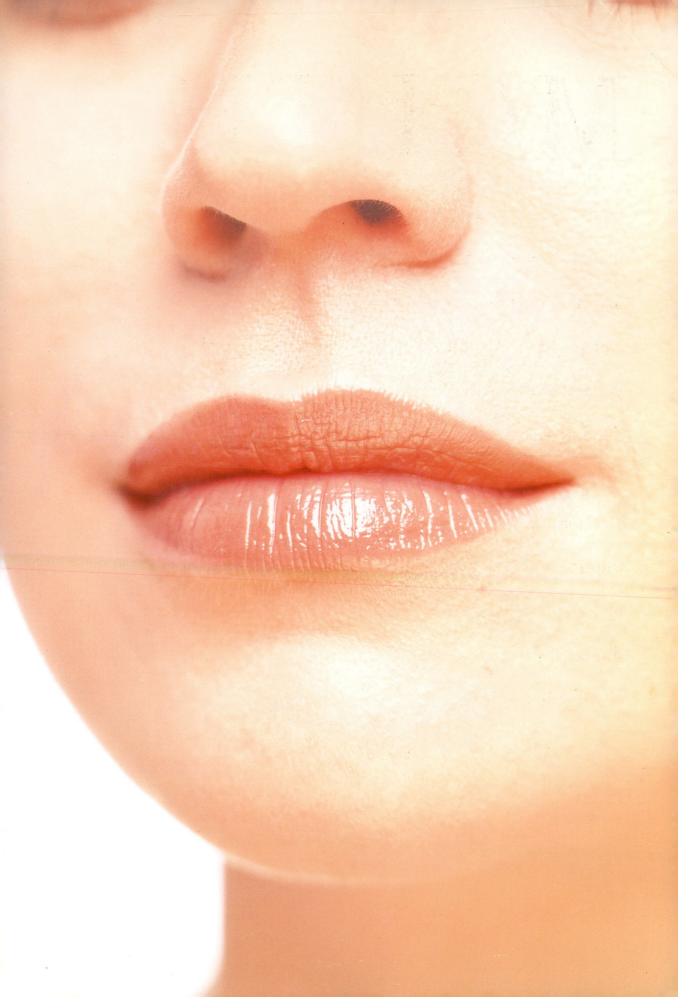

LIPS & MOUTH

Care of the mouth and scrupulous oral hygiene are necessary for beauty care. Because we use our mouths to communicate, eat, and kiss, they are of importance to the sensory system. Brush your teeth thoroughly morning and evening, but take care not to overbrush as this can cause gum erosion that leads to problems later in life. Try to use a toothpaste that is based on natural ingredients rather than synthetics. If your water supply does not contain added fluoride, choose a toothpaste that contains fluoride but check with your dentist on how often to use it. To exfoliate your lips, use an old dry toothbrush, then apply lip balm.

Preparations for lips and mouth

Fruit and Nut Lip Salve

The peanut oil with its infusion of raspberry and strawberry leaves tightens and smooths, making a good base for lipstick.

Ingredients

2 tsp (10 ml) strawberry leaves

2 tbsp (30 ml) raspberry leaves

2 tbsp (30 ml) beeswax

2 tsp (10 ml) peanut oil

To make

Cover the leaves with a small amount of hot (not boiling) water and leave to infuse for at least a few hours. Heat the beeswax in a small bowl over simmering water. Add the peanut oil gradually and mix thoroughly, to a thick paste consistency. You may not need all the oil. Strain the infusion and mix in some liquid, using enough to achieve a thin paste consistency. Put into a small jar and store in the refrigerator to solidify.

To use

Apply to the lips. You can lightly exfoliate the lips with an old toothbrush before applying the softening balm.

Coconut Lip Balm

A coconut oil base with soothing chickweed herb helps to counteract chapped lips.

Ingredients

2 tbsp (30 ml) coconut oil

1 tsp (5 ml) chickweed tincture

Chickweed flowers to decorate

To make

Heat the coconut oil in a small bowl over hot water. Add the tincture and stir. Place the flowers in the bottom of a small clear glass jar, pour the oil on top and leave in a cool place to set.

To use

Apply to the lips.

Tea Tree, Lavender and Geranium Cold Sore Remedy

For cold sores, this is effective and antibacterial. It helps to prevent repeat infections, as tea tree oil boosts the immune system.

Ingredients

2 tbsp (30 ml) vodka

2 tbsp (30 ml) warm water

2 drops tea tree essential oil

2 drops geranium essential oil

2 drops lavender essential oil

5 drops echinacea tincture

1 tsp (5 ml) whole milk

To make

Mix all the ingredients together. The alcohol preserves the milk, which disperses the oil in the liquids. Echinacea helps prevent infections and counteracts boils.

To use

Dab on the affected areas, using a cotton swab so you do not introduce bacteria onto the cold sore. (Do not re-use the cotton swab.) Cold sores are caused by a virus, so cannot be cured, but this remedy will help if you catch them early enough.

Mandarin Mouthwash

For those who dislike the taste of mint, generally the flavoring of most oral hygiene products, this cleanses and freshens the breath.

Ingredients

2 tbsp (30 ml) warm water

2 drops mandarin essential oil

2 drops whole milk

To make

Mix all the ingredients together. The milk helps the oil disperse.

To use

Do not swallow the essential oil. For children use only 1 drop of essential oil. Never take essential oil internally.

tooth powder, wash and rinse

Baking Soda Tooth Powder

This is extremely effective for cleaning teeth and leaves the mouth tingling. It contains dried banana powder for flavor and gum nourishment.

Ingredients

2 tbsp (30 ml) baking soda
2 tsp (10 ml) dried banana flour (powder)
2 drops peppermint essential oil

To make

Mix all the ingredients together. Dried banana powder is not always easy to find, but you may get it from Asian supermarkets or wholesalers. Add the essential oil and mix to the consistency of fine breadcrumbs.

To use

Dampen the toothbrush, place some powder on it and use as usual. The toothpaste will not foam, as it contains no detergent, but this does not make it any less effective.

Cinnamon and Calendula Mouthwash

Made from an extract of calendula flowers, this mouthwash is strongly antifungal.

Ingredients

3 tbsp (45 ml) calendula flowers
2 tbsp (30 ml) warm water
1 stick cinnamon bark (about 2 in/ 5 cm), broken into small pieces
1 tsp (5 ml) vodka
1 drop peppermint essential oil (optional)
1 tsp (5 ml) milk (optional)

To make

Combine the calendula flowers and the warm water, leave to infuse for about five to ten minutes. Make sure the water is not boiling as this will blanch the flowers and some of the healing properties will be lost. Strain the infusion and add the cinnamon to the liquid. Leave this to infuse at least overnight, then strain to remove the cinnamon and add the vodka.

To use

Swish around the mouth as usual. You may add a drop of peppermint essential oil and a dash of milk to make this mouthwash stronger, but do not substitute cinnamon essential oil for the bark, as it is extremely strong and may be toxic if taken internally.

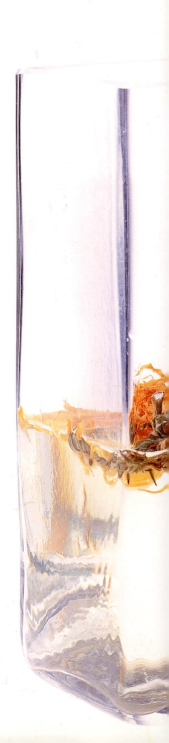

Parsley Oil Mouth Rinse

A traditional odor remover, parsley is also antifungal and so prevents infection and mouth ulcers.

Ingredients

2 tbsp (30 ml) water

1 tsp (5 ml) whole milk

2 drops parsley essential oil

To make

Mix all the ingredients together.

To use

Swish around the mouth as usual. Do not swallow the mouthwash, as essential oils should not be taken internally without guidance.

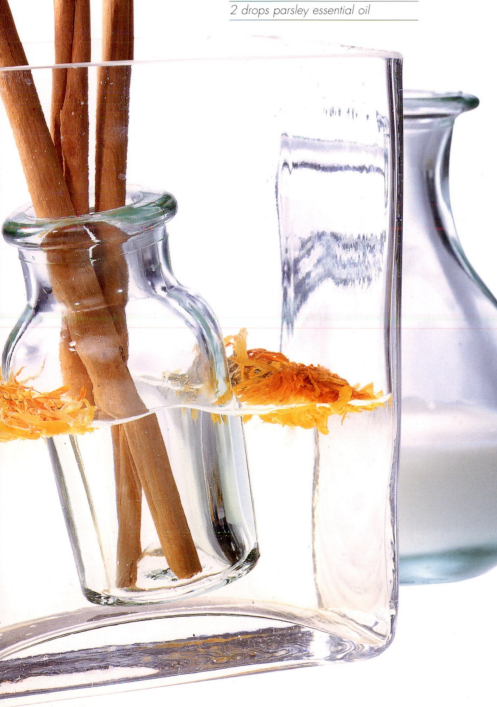

BATHING

Bathing is an ancient tradition, dating back to ancient Egypt and later the Roman spas. Relaxing and reviving, a bath can be the ultimate in "time out." Athletic men and women often have a warm bath to relax the muscles after intense exercise and, in the case of gymnasts, it can even improve flexibility. Overly hot water can have an adverse effect, however, and make you feel sluggish and even dizzy in extreme cases. The advantage of using essential oils and other bath preparations is that the water helps them evaporate and become more effective. Also, the skin is more absorbent when warm and moist. Applying lotions after bathing is a great way to seal in moisture, especially for people with dry skin. A bath can be a great opportunity for a head-to-toe beauty treat.

As with the shampoos, some of these recipes use a base that has been purchased and not made. Again, you can make your own base, but it tends to be tricky and it is especially difficult to make a foaming base. It is fairly easy to buy dispersing bath base, either in oil or bubble form.

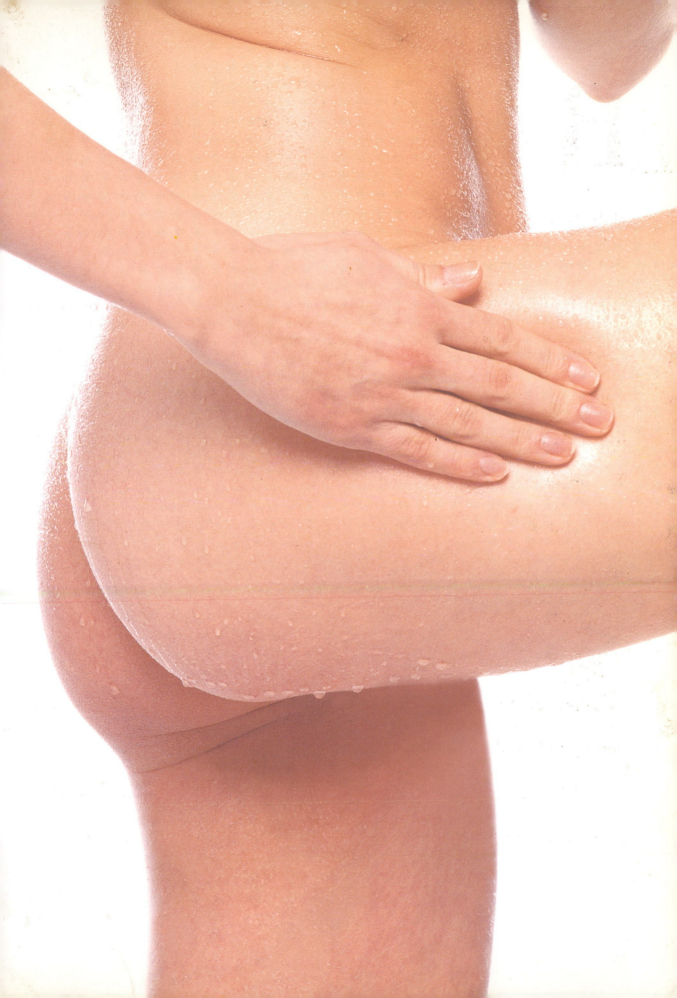

BATHTIME

Bathing is a wonderful way to relax. In summer time, for a refreshing and invigorating treat, add some rosemary to a cool bath. When the weather is colder, a hot bath with eucalyptus or thyme oil will warm the skin and leave it glowing. Thyme oil helps to boost the immunity so it is especially helpful during outbreaks of colds and influenza. Brushing the skin with a coarse body brush while taking a bath is a good way to exfoliate. The warm water, combined with a brushing motion, brings blood to the surface of the skin and produces a rejuvenating effect. If you use soap on the brush at the same time, your skin will be squeaky clean.

bath additions

Honey and Lemon Bath Elixir

Mild and soothing, yet uplifting, this preparation leaves the skin silky smooth and pampered—a perfect start for an evening out.

Ingredients

2 tbsp (30 ml) runny honey

2 tbsp (30 ml) fresh lemon juice

2 tbsp (30 ml) bath base
(oil or bubbles)

To make

Fold the honey and lemon juice into the bath base slowly and thoroughly. The dispersing base helps the honey dissolve in the bath. You can substitute milk, but you will get no bubbles and you will need very warm water to dissolve the honey.

To use

The large proportion of honey makes this recipe very rich, and you only need to pour a small amount under running water to create a luxurious bath. If your base oil has a detergent added (often sold as "bubbling base oil"), you will have soft, scented bubbles in your bath.

Rose Milk Bath

It is pure indulgence to spend hours in a bath of rose petals, milk and rose oil. Rose oil can be expensive, but it is worth treating yourself to a small bottle for use on special occasions.

Ingredients

3 drops rose essential oil

2 tbsp (30 ml) whole milk

2 tbsp (30 ml) fresh or dried rose
petals (for decoration)

To make

You may either use rose absolute oil or rose otto (usually slightly cheaper). The absolute is premium quality, so be careful when dispensing it to avoid waste; it can take up to 125 pounds (57 kg) of rose petals to produce a 1-ounce (30 ml) bottle of rose absolute essential oil. Combine the milk, oil and petals and store in a clear jar. This bath elixir looks lovely displayed on a bathroom shelf and will keep for a few weeks in a cool place.

To use

Pour a small amount under running water.

Raspberry Bubbles

Fun and energizing, this recipe doubles as a shower gel for speedy washing.

Ingredients

2 tbsp (30 ml) bath base (oil or bubbles)

1 cup (about 8 oz/225 g) fresh raspberries

1 drop tea tree essential oil

To make

Try to buy a thick consistency base soap so the end result is not too runny. Use a blender to whiz all the ingredients together, or alternatively, purée the raspberries and then mix in the other ingredients, ensuring the oil is thoroughly dispersed. Refrigerate overnight to set and store in the refrigerator after use. Due to the fresh fruit and lack of preservative, this recipe will not last more than about a week, so don't make a large amount.

To use

Pour a small amount under running bath water, or use as a shower gel.

BATH SALTS

All the bath salts are made in the same way, with different ingredients added for fragrance and to give them various properties. Epsom salts are very good for the skin, drawing out impurities and locking in moisture.

bath additions

Basic Bath Salts Mixture

Ingredients

3 tbsp (45 ml) Epsom salts
1 tbsp (15 ml) orris root
1 tsp (5 ml) cornstarch (corn flour)

Variations

1) Add two drops of lavender essential oil and two drops of geranium essential oil for a relaxing and balancing bath.

2) Add two drops of sandalwood essential oil and two tablespoons of baking soda for a fizzy and exotic bath.

3) Add some rose and marigold petals for a pretty, gently fragrant bath that will soften the skin.

To make

Mix all the ingredients, along with a selection from the variations above. If you are adding essential oil, make sure it is thoroughly dispersed. Cornstarch softens the skin and holds the other ingredients together. The orris root softens and helps retain the fragrance in the bath salts; it may also make them solidify a little over time, but this is not a concern.

To use

Add a small handful of salts to your bath.

Geranium and Orange Bath Salts

Ingredients

3 tbsp (45 ml) Epsom salts
1 tbsp (15 ml) orris root
1 tbsp (15 ml) dried orange peel
1 tbsp (15ml) dried orange flowers
1 drop orange essential oil
3 drops geranium essential oil

To make

Mix all the ingredients, thoroughly dispersing the essential oil in the salt. This bath salt does not contain cornstarch because the orange peel and flowers already give it the texture needed. You can buy dried orange peel and flowers, or you can dry orange slices yourself by heating in a very hot oven then transferring to a warm cupboard for at least two weeks. The heat from the oven seals in moisture and prevents molding, but do check after about a week for any signs of mold. If this happens, discard the orange and start again. Dried orange slices make a fragrant addition to potpourri or to a Chrismas decoration.

To use

Add a small handful of salts to your bath.

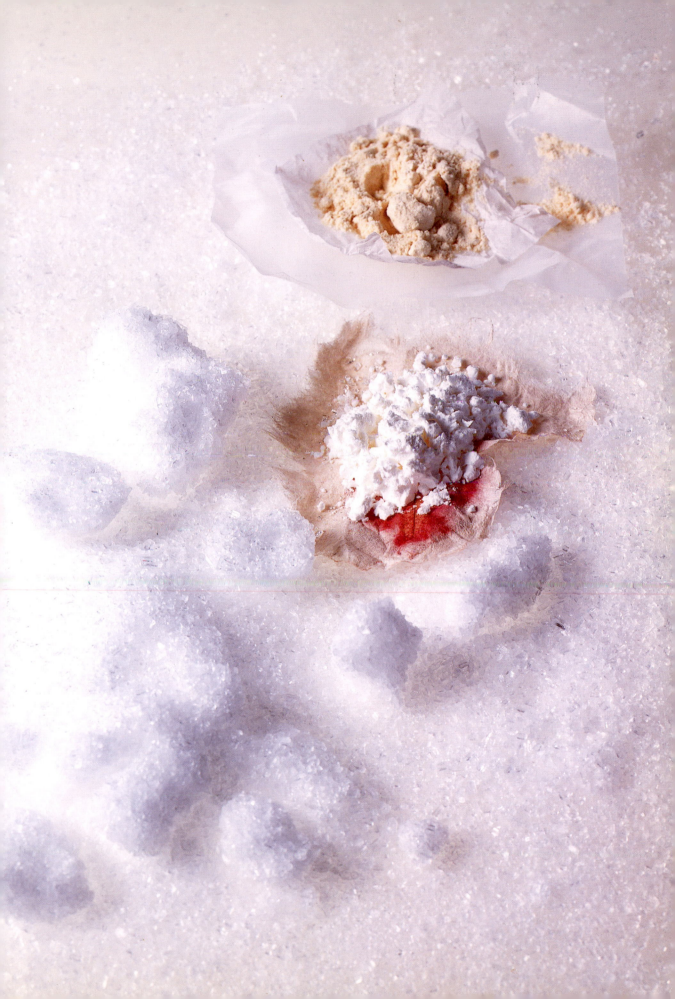

SOAPS

Making your own soap is well worth the effort. Liquid soap is the easiest to begin with if you are new to making your own beauty preparations. Soaps are less messy and difficult to make than bases for shampoos or bath preparations, as soap needs only to solidify and not to disperse. Also, if you go wrong it is easy to add more liquid or solid ingredients. In fact, all the quantities here are fairly flexible, as they will depend on the quality of your raw ingredients and the speed with which you make the soap. You will need to experiment a little before you get correct consistencies. These soaps will foam less than commercial soaps, as they have no chemical additions, but the baking soda makes them cleansing.

making soap

To set a soap

Exact instructions on soap making are included in the relevant recipes. However, there are two tips I would add for making up any solid preparation, such as a soap or moisture bar. It is a good idea to pour part of the liquid in the mold and allow it to set before pouring more in. This will create a layered bar and have the advantage of making the soap stronger. You can place fruit or anything you wish to set in the soap in the mold halfway through this process to ensure it is thoroughly embedded and does not rise to the surface or sink to the bottom.

In addition, using cookie cutters is an excellent way of making shaped novelty soaps, and is especially good for children.

Rose Geranium Liquid Soap

Convenient to use and easy to make, try keeping it in a pump-top dispenser for easy access. Geranium has a gentle, invigorating fragrance.

Ingredients

1 tbsp (15 ml) rose water
2 tbsp (30 ml) baking soda
2 drops rose oil
2 drops geranium oil
2 tbsp (30 ml) aloe vera gel

To make

Warm the rose water and dissolve the baking soda in it. Cool until lukewarm, then add the essential oils (not before or they will evaporate). Fold in the aloe vera gel and refrigerate overnight to chill completely.

To use

Particularly good for dry skin. Use as normal soap.

Petitgrain and Bois de Rose Deodorizing Soap

Great for hot days, this is a good recipe for sweaty feet. These two oils have strong deodorizing properties and combine well in a soap.

Ingredients

1 tbsp (15 ml) sweet almond oil
2 drops petitgrain essential oil
2 drops bois de rose essential oil
3 tbsp (45 ml) baking soda
1 tbsp (15 ml) beeswax
3 tbsp (45 ml) glycerin

To make

Warm the almond oil and essential oils in a small bowl over simmering water. Add the baking soda, stirring vigorously until dissolved (be patient and do not overheat the oil or it will start spitting). Next, keeping the water heated, add the beeswax. Stir until melted and thoroughly mixed with the other ingredients. Last, add the glycerin and beat all the ingredients together with a fork over the hot water until well combined. Pour into a small bowl or mold lined with parchment paper and refrigerate overnight to set.

Check the soap; it should be solid. If it is not, reheat and add more glycerin (using the method above). If it is too hard, reheat and add more oil. You can do this a couple of times before the ingredients denature and have to be thrown away.

To use

Use as a normal soap, but do not let it float in a warm bath, as it will melt quickly. Best stored in the refrigerator.

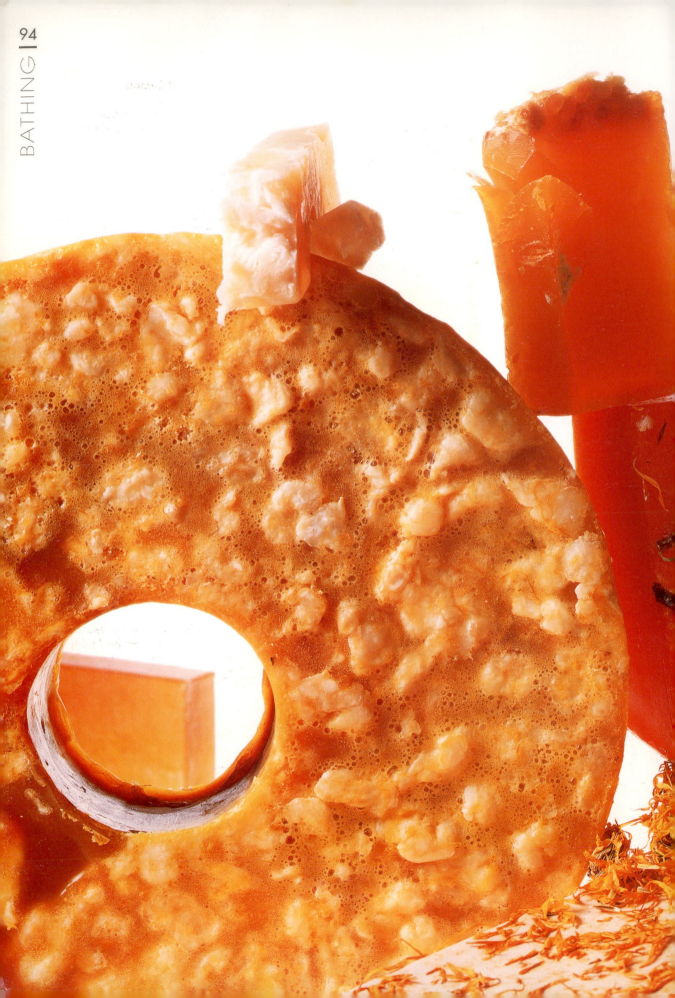

Orange and Lemon Glycerin Soap

This contains slices of whole lemon and orange. Softening and sweet, it smells heavenly.

Ingredients

3 lemon slices, about ¼ inch (5 mm) thick, halved
3 orange slices, about ¼ inch (5 mm) thick, halved
1 tbsp (15 ml) sweet almond oil
1 drop lemon essential oil
1 drop orange essential oil
3 tbsp (45 ml) baking soda
1 tbsp (15 ml) beeswax
3 tbsp (45 ml) glycerin

To make

Put the lemon and orange slices to one side. Combine the remaining ingredients in exactly the same way as the Petitgrain and Bois de Rose Deodorizing Soap (see page 92). Once the soap is heated and fully mixed, pour half into the paper-lined bowl or mold. Place the lemon and orange slices on the soap surface, keeping the remaining half of the soap mixture warm. Now pour the remaining soap over the fruit, and leave to set in the refrigerator.

To use

The fruit is mainly for decoration; however, the peel adds some astringent properties to the soap.

BODY LOTIONS

Moisturizing the body after showering or bathing is a great way to lightly perfume the skin, lock in moisture and protect dry skin. A base lotion is used, which may be obtained easily from any herbalist or apothecary. Be sure to use a base with no added synthetics or fragrance. Equally, you can make your own base lotion as described.

body moisturizers

Base lotion

Essential oils can be added to this base for homemade cosmetics. Those with more sensitive skin can use it alone.

Ingredients

1 tbsp (15 ml) lanolin
3 tbsp (45 ml) sweet almond oil
1 tbsp (15 ml) aloe vera gel

To make

Lanolin is a naturally occurring oily substance appearing on sheep's wool. You can find it easily at a pharmacy. Mix the almond oil and aloe vera gel thoroughly in a small bowl. Place the bowl over simmering water and melt the lanolin, stirring it in with the other ingredients. Remove from the heat and beat until the mixture has cooled. Transfer to a jar.

To use

Apply as any moisturizer to the body or face.

Rose Moisturizer for Mature Skin

This provides gentle fragrance and deep conditioning.

Ingredients

2 drops liquid vitamin E
2 drops rose essential oil
4 tbsp (60 ml) base lotion
1 tsp (5 ml) rose water

To make

Add the vitamin E and essential oil, little by little, to the base lotion, stirring to mix. You may not need the rose water if your lotion is quite thin. The vitamin E will make the lotion yellow in color; do not be concerned.

To use

Apply as a normal moisturizer, especially on the face.

Apricot Rough Skin Lotion

This provides super moisture for dry areas such as elbows and knees.

Ingredients

3 tbsp (45 ml) base lotion
1 tbsp (15 ml) ground apricot kernels
1 tsp (5 ml) apricot kernel oil

To make

Simply mix all ingredients together until well combined.

To use

Apply as a normal moisturizer and rub the apricot lotion into the skin to exfoliate, then brush off when the lotion has been absorbed and dried.

Camomile and Calendula Dry Skin Cream

Good to treat mild eczema and dry skin conditions. Do not substitute tinctures of camomile and calendula, as the alcohol in these is too drying.

Ingredients

2 tbsp (30 ml) camomile flowers
2 tbsp (30 ml) calendula petals
2 tbsp (30 ml) base lotion

To make

Cover the camomile and calendula flowers with hot (not boiling) water and leave to infuse (see page 15). When cooled, strain and mix some of the liquid into the base lotion. Use as much as necessary to produce a loose-consistency lotion; you will not need all.

To use

Apply normally. Especially good on dry, rough areas. Suitable for use on the face.

PERFUMING

Commercial deodorants work by blocking the sweat producing pores and preventing perspiration. Long-term use has a harsh effect on the skin. Even some of the more natural deodorants are potentially harmful— some deodorant crystals are actually almost solid aluminum. Your body adapts to natural fragrance and does not produce more perspiration to counteract the blocking effect of commercial products. It is possible to make your own deodorant and scent from natural products. Other homemade fragrances include potpourri and room fresheners, which revive the senses and leave any space filled with a lovely scent.

There are a few basic rules about blending fragrances. Scents are mainly split into three categories, and in any perfume you need to combine them carefully to not overemphasize one type of fragrance.

The top note provides the lingering sweetest fragrance. The middle note rounds out the fragrance, creating depth. The base notes are often the underlying fragrance of a perfume. These fragrances fix the overall scent. For a sweeter fragrance, use more than one top note; a more musky fragrance is achieved with the emphasis on the middle notes; for a heavier, more masculine fragrance, concentrate on the base notes.

THE BODY

TOILET WATERS

Toilet waters are a traditional way to fragrance the skin, and are especially good to use after a bath when the skin is soft and absorbs more moisture. You can also use them as a room fragrance (dispensed from a pump-action spray bottle), and to fragrance fresh laundry, (unlike essential oils, they will not stain). Very high quality orange flower water is used in cooking, and rose water is an essential ingredient in many Middle Eastern recipes.

making fragrances

Eucalyptus, Thyme and Tea Tree Deodorant Spray

Strong and antibacterial, this preparation has a light non-clogging alcohol base.

Ingredients

3 tbsp (45 ml) vodka
3 tbsp (45 ml) distilled water
2 drops tea tree essential oil
2 drops thyme essential oil
2 drops eucalyptus essential oil

To make
Combine all the ingredients in a spray-top bottle.

To use
Shake well to disperse the oil. Spray on the underarms as needed.

Rosewood Solid Deodorant

Soda crystals are mixed with this excellent deodorizing plant extract. Extremely effective, it may be rubbed all over the body, especially the underarms.

Ingredients

1 cup (240 ml) baking soda
2 drops bois de rose essential oil
1 tbsp (15 ml) rosewood herb

To make
Add a small amount of water to the baking soda and mix with your fingertips until it is the consistency of breadcrumbs. Do not add too much water, or the mixture will become sticky. Mix with the remaining ingredients. Store in a cool place, in a screw-top jar, to seal in fragrance.

To use
This deodorant is powdery in consistency. Use by rubbing a small amount into the underarms after bathing. Make sure the underarm is dry before use or the powder will clog; also, baking soda reacts with moisture.

Natural Eau de Cologne

A toilet water of alcohol base, contains oils of petitgrain, cedarwood, bergamot and orange.

Ingredients

3 tbsp (45 ml) vodka
3 tbsp (45 ml) distilled water
2 drops petitgrain essential oil
2 drops cedarwood essential oil
2 drops bergamot essential oil
2 drops orange essential oil

To make
Mix all ingredients together in a spray- top bottle.

To use
Shake well to disperse the oil. Spray on the underarms as needed.

Lavender Water

Made with lavender flowers in a distilled water base, it is light, refreshing and traditional.

Ingredients

2 tbsp (30 ml) lavender flowers (dried or fresh)
3 tbsp (45 ml) distilled water
1 tsp (5 ml) vodka
2 drops lavender essential oil (optional)

To make
Leave the flowers to infuse in a sealed bottle in the water and alcohol for at least twenty four hours, or up to a week. If you would like the water to be a little stronger in fragrance, add the lavender essential oil. Strain and bottle the liquid.

To use
Shake the bottle before use, especially if you added the essential oil. Use as a perfume or light deodorant.

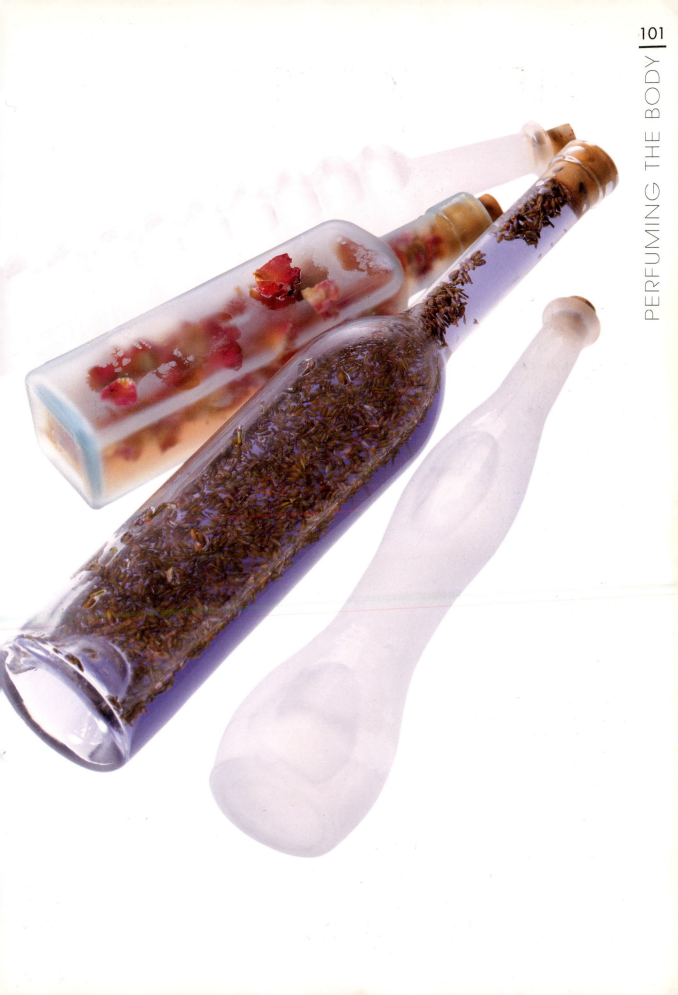

toilet waters and potpourri

Jasmine and Cornflower Toilet Water

This is rich, exotic and indulgent.

Ingredients

2 tbsp (30 ml) cornflowers (dried or fresh)
3 tbsp (45 ml) distilled water
1 tsp (5 ml) vodka
2 drops jasmine essential oil

To make

Jasmine essential oil can be very expensive, but is well worth the investment. It is reputedly a useful remedy for stress and the early stages of flu, as well as having a heady and exotic fragrance. It is possible to buy a synthetic jasmine fragrance, but I would not recommend this. Cornflowers are also a slightly unusual ingredient. You may find them sold as an ingredient for making potpourri. Many people have cornflowers growing in their gardens. Leave the cornflowers to infuse in the water and alcohol for three hours (not much longer as they become soggy and there is little advantage in this). Strain and add the jasmine essential oil to the liquid.

To use

Shake the bottle before use to disperse the essential oil. Use as a perfume or light deodorant.

Sandalwood Toilet Water

Woody and heavy, this is especially suitable for men.

Ingredients

3 tbsp (45 ml) distilled water
1 tsp (5 ml) vodka
3 drops sandalwood essential oil
1 drop cedarwood oil

To make

Mix all the ingredients together, in a spray-top bottle.

To use

Shake well to disperse the oil. Spray on the underarms as needed.

Lavender Flower Potpourri

This potpourri is a traditional mixture.

Ingredients

3 drops lavender essential oil

2 tsp (10 ml) orris root

3 tbsp (45 ml) fresh lavender flowers

To make

Using a spoon, mix the lavender oil with the orris root in a bowl. Add the flowers and mix again. Put the mixture in a plastic bag, seal and leave in a warm place for at least a month and up to three months.

To use

Display in an open container and revive with essential oil if necessary.

Spicy Potpourri

A lovely room freshener, this is warming and smells like Christmas.

Ingredients

2 drops orange essential oil

1 tbsp (15 ml) orris root

1 tbsp (15 ml) lavender flowers

2 sticks cinnamon bark
  (about 2 in/5 cm), broken
    into small pieces

1 crushed nutmeg

6 small pine cones

1 tbsp (15 ml) fresh calendula petals

1 tbsp (15 ml) fresh rose petals

To make

Mix the essential oil with the orris root in a bowl, using a spoon to avoid getting the essential oil on your hands. Combine with all the other ingredients, thoroughly mixed, in a plastic bag. Seal the bag and leave in a warm place for at least a month and up to three months; the potpourri needs time to mature.

To use

Display in a pretty dish. You can revive the fragrance by adding more essential oil later. The potpourri will best perfume a small area such as a bathroom, as the fragrance is lost in larger areas.

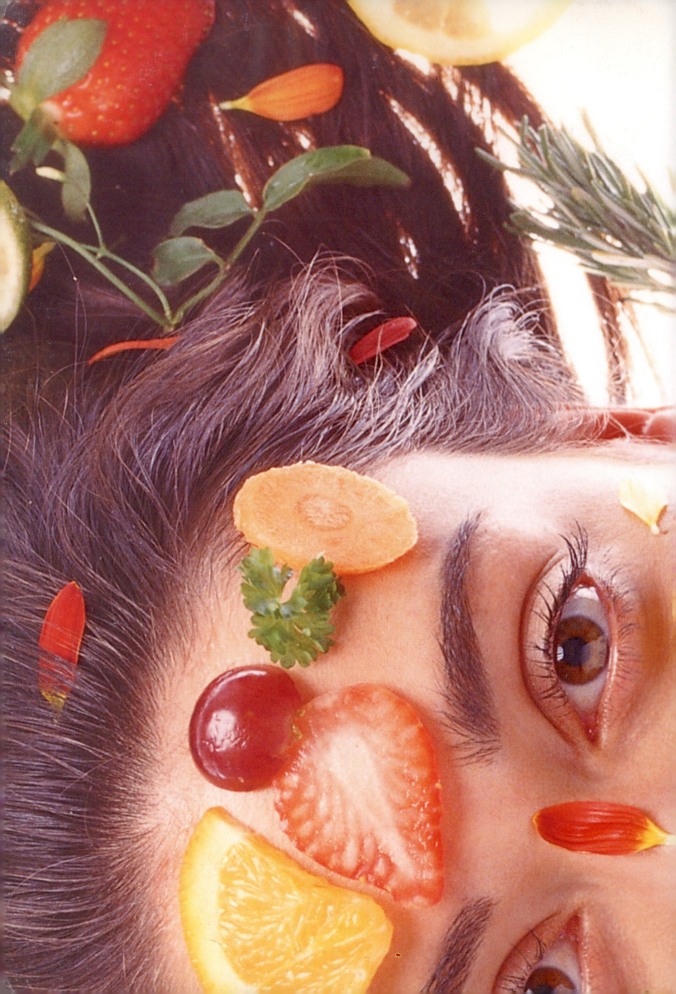

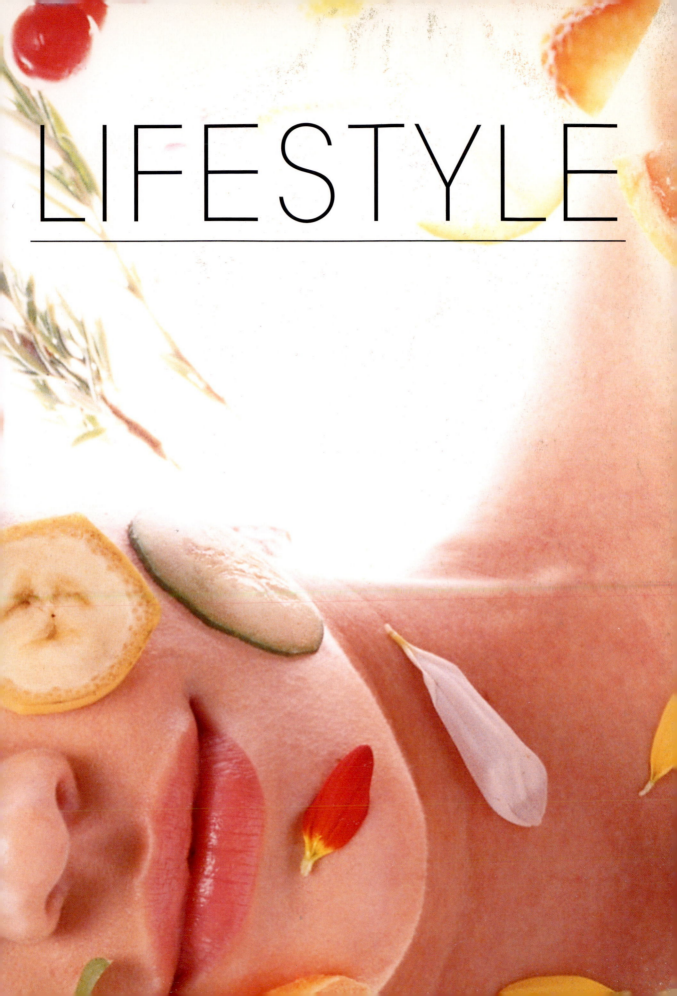

LIFESTYLE

MASSAGE

Massage is one of the most ancient healing arts. Dating from the times of ancient Greek and Roman civilizations, massage is unique in its ability to nurture, heal and enrich health. Massage works by stimulating our sense of touch and smell. Fragrances are the first stimulus of any to be registered by the brain, so the effect of aromatic essential oils is instant as well as long lasting. The importance of touch is often underestimated in today's rushed world of technology and machines. Nothing can replace old-fashioned human touch. In cancer patients for example, studies have shown that massage can help with associated anxiety and even aids patients in accepting and understanding the changes going on in their bodies.

Top note	Middle note	Bottom note
tea tree	lavender	patchouli
eucalyptus	marjoram	rose
mandarin	rosewood	jasmine
basil	rosemary	benzoin
lemon	geranium	frankincense
lemongrass	palma rosa	myrrh

A combination of top notes, middle notes and bottom notes are blended to make a massage oil with a balanced fragrance.

Self-massage helps us connect with our bodies and our own health; massaging another person is a way of communicating and spending time with a friend or relation. Massage offers the following benefits:

- deepens relaxation.
- improves circulation.
- stimulates lymphatic system, boosting immunity.
- aids digestion, speeds the elimination of toxins.
- improves skin circulation and quality.
- increases blood supply to joints, can help arthritis.
- relieves mental and physical fatigue.

The Role of Oils

The scent of aromatherapy oils enters the brain via the olfactory neurons. Information then moves to a specialized part of the brain that connects the fragrance with memory, feelings and emotions. In this way certain smells may be a very strong anchor (memory stimulus) to certain situations or emotions. It is important that when you use essential oils you actually like the fragrances you are using; otherwise you may find they are less effective and even unpleasant.

A further way essential oils can enter the system is via the skin, directly into the blood supply. The usual application in this case is by massaging essential oils diluted in plain base oils directly into the skin. One or two drops of oils in the bath, dispersed with a dash of fatty milk, also have direct results. Never apply undiluted essential oils neat onto the skin or in the bath without a dispersing agent, as they will burn the skin.

It is important to always take the advice of a trained practitioner or doctor where relevant. Massage and aromatherapy are complementary to and not a replacement for other treatments. Do not try selftreatment during pregnancy or during periods of long-term or serious illness. For safe use, observe the following guidelines:

- keep essential oils away from pets and children.
- never take essential oils internally.
- never apply essential oils directly on to the skin, except in the case of lavender or tea tree oil in small quantities.
- during pregnancy consult an aromatherapist before using essential oils. Mandarin, however is usually safe (in France it is known as "the child's oil").
- dilute oils well for use on sensitive skin.
- store oils in dark glass bottles in a cool place. Do not leave rubber droppers in the oil as it will cause them to disintegrate and may denature the oil.

Certain essential oils may help to counteract negative emotions, because they trigger a positive emotional reaction. For example, camomile and frankincense are joyful, lighthearted fragrances that moderate feelings of anger. Essential oils also have a physiological effect as they are absorbed via the skin or nasal passages into the blood stream, but these effects may be milder.

Massage is easily learned and with a little practice may be administered by anyone. Even children can learn massage. It is important to set up suitable conditions in which to learn and develop your massage skills. Make sure you and your massage partner will not be disturbed. There is little worse than being disturbed by a ringing phone or doorbell while trying to create an atmosphere of relaxation and nurturing. Soft, pleasant music may enhance the atmosphere and aid relaxation. You will need several warm towels of varying sizes. If your partner needs extra support, for example under the head or knee, use a rolled up small towel. You will also need a surface from which to work.

A massage couch may be used, but these tend to be expensive. I prefer to work from the floor on a futon or even a comfortable camping mattress covered with towels. As well as providing warmth and comfort, the towels protect surfaces from oil.

For your own comfort it is important to wear loose clothes and make sure you are warm enough. Remember that as your partner relaxes, his or her body temperature will lower, so he or she may feel colder than you.

Starting your Massage

The most important part of any massage is the initial touch. Quality of touch is the key here. Gently slide your hands onto your partner, having warmed and oiled them slightly. Gradually add more oil until you have a smooth surface of skin to work with (not too oily or you will be sliding all over the place). I suggest the best place to start massaging is the back, as it is the largest surface area of the body.

emotion	Useful oils
anger	camomile, frankincense, grapefruit
depression	geranium, rosemary, bergamot
grief	marjoram, clary sage, bergamot
indecision	cedar, peppermint, grapefruit
insomnia	frankincense, lavender, clary sage
jealousy	sandlewood, palma rosa, myrrh
negativity	juniper, neroli, bergamot
sadness	coriander, pine, rosemary
stress	basil, geranium, rosemary

BACK MASSAGE

1) Position your friend lying on his or her front and sit yourself by their side. Apply some oil to your hands and gently apply to your friend's back. Cover the body below the waist with a warm towel. Apply the oil in a sweeping motion across the whole back. Remember to be gentle but firm.

2) Knead the shoulder and hip area with a side-to-side movement and pick up areas of flesh as you sweep down the sides of the body. This stroke loosens the muscle and very gently eases tight muscle from the bone.

3) Now you can start to work across the muscle groups. This stroke is known as wringing: pull your whole hand across the back and push smoothly back.

4) Once the area is looser and warm you may start to work more deeply. Imagine the back muscles are a lump of butter. Start by working into specific tense areas, then as the muscle loosens and "melts," work in deeper. Never hurt your friend and always ask if the pressure is comfortable. As you practice massage you will soon become able to detect areas of built up tension.

5) You can now soothe the areas you have just worked on with some circling strokes. Place one hand on top of the other to do this.

6) Finish with a broad stroke to make the massage feel complete and lastly feather the back with soft, light fingers.

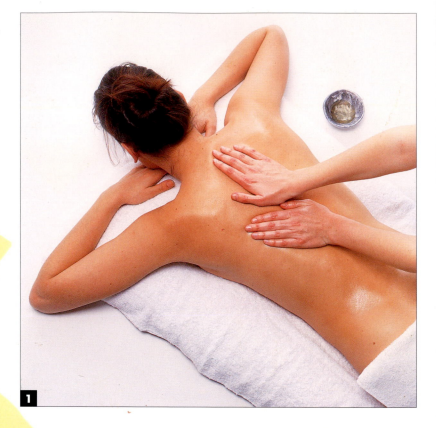

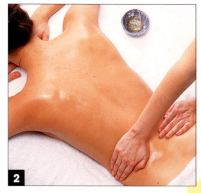

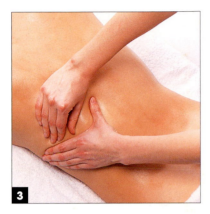

3

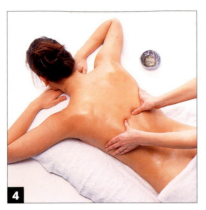

4

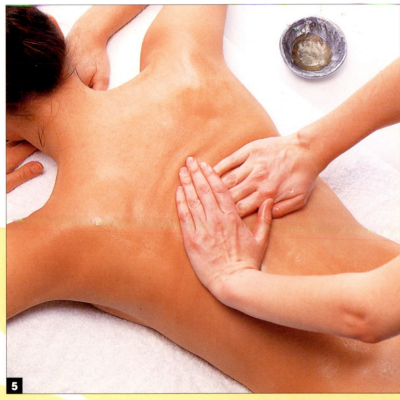

5

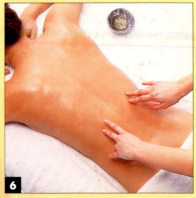

6

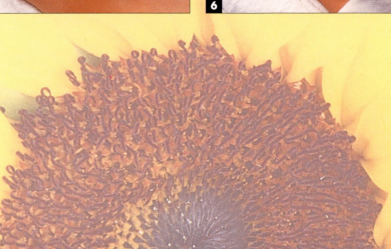

FACIAL MASSAGE

Give yourself or a friend a facial. You may either use aromatherapy oils or use your favorite beauty products (try a face mask followed by exfoliation, then apply your moisturizer with massage strokes). Facial massage is a great way of toning facial muscles and keeping the skin tight and firm. The face contains more muscles than any part of the body, and although the old saying of the wind changing to fix a grumpy face in place for ever is not true, smiling does help counteract facial wrinkles, as well as stimulating the thymus gland and boosting immunity.

1) Make sure your friend's neck is well supported and not overstretched. Sit behind your friend's head.

2) It is very important to lower the hands onto the face very gently, as it is very unpleasant to have heavy hands placed on your face. Remember how sensitive the face is.

3a) Gently stroke your thumbs across the forehead. 3b) Stroke the thumbs down the cheeks. 3c) Pull the thumbs up over the chin. Turn the rest of your hands away from your friend's face.

4) Gently pinch the chin in an upward motion. This stroke helps to prevent a double chin.

5) Using a light tapping motion, cover the face in gentle "raindrops." This stroke invigorates and brings blood to the surface of the skin, improving circulation.

6) Finish by gently cupping your hands over your friend's eyes and holding them there for a while. Ask your friend to take a deep breath and allow him or her a moment to relax.

7) Finish by gently stroking your hands through your friend's hair.

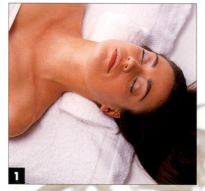

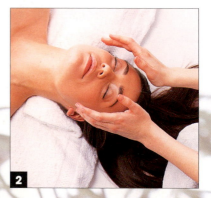

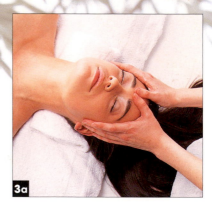

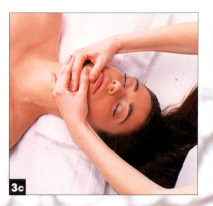

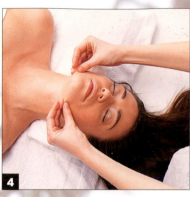

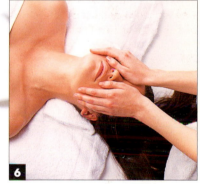

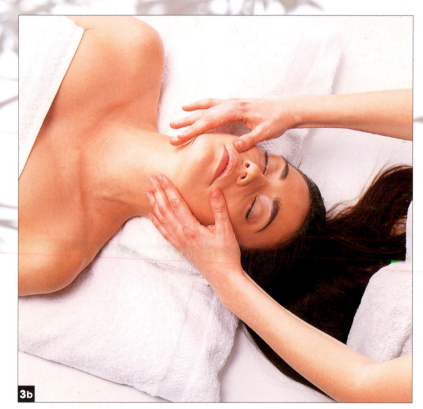

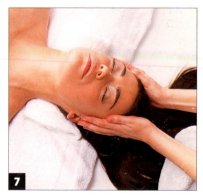

DIET

For most people a healthful diet means one containing plenty of fruit and vegetables, some fiber, and not too many sweets and high-fat foods. Given enough time and effort, it is possible to create a diet that is so healthy and nutritious that it satisfies all our vitamin and mineral requirements, a diet of true optimum nutrition. However, most of us find we need some carefully selected vitamin and mineral supplements in addition to our daily diet to achieve this level of optimum health.

As far as weight management is concerned, it is not only the traditional counting of calories that is important, even when considered in conjunction with exercise. Scientists and top nutritionists are now discovering that metabolism is perhaps the most important factor in how our bodies assimilate and process food. Metabolism is the process of turning food into either energy or fat. For most of us, usually most of the time the former is preferable. Foods that are least likely to be stored as fat are slow-release carbohydrates (lentils, beans, vegetables, whole grains). Fruit may be eaten if a quick energy fix is required, because although it contains sugar, it is in the form of fructose, which does not "shock" the blood sugar system nearly as much as glucose (normal sugar) and so is less likely to be stored as fat.

WONDER FOODS

Although most fruits and vegetables are nutritious and healthy, some are truly wonder foods—foods that are actively good for the system and help create maximum health and vitality. The importance of an organic diet is immense. In one year on average we breathe in 0.07 ounce (2 grams) of solid pollution, eat 12 pounds (5.5 kilograms) of food additives, and consume some 6,000 chemicals via our food intake, not to mention the gallons of pesticides sprayed onto the fruit and vegetables we eat. Although for fiber content it is better to eat the skins of fruit and vegetables, these days you may be taking in more harm than good. All these chemicals break down the immune system, cause premature aging and have been linked with medical conditions such as heart disease and cancer. Bearing these facts in mind, when purchasing fruit and vegetables or for making the preparations in this book, think organic.

Foods for health and vitality

Oats
Oats are one of the few internationally accepted foods that have active benefits for your health. Oats actively lower cholesterol. Eating a bowl of oatmeal in the morning is a great way to start the day. A slow-releasing carbohydrate, oats will provide long-lasting energy over a period of time.

Sunflower
Sunflower oil is vegetable-based, and one of the few vegetarian fat sources. It provides lots of vitamin E, which the World Health Organization suggests is important in preventing heart attack. Sunflower seeds are rich in antioxidants, which are thought to have anti-cancer properties.

Grapefruit

Grapefruit subtly increases the body's metabolism, so it promotes fat burning and is great to eat after a meal. Citrus fruit has been linked with reducing the likelihood of developing cancer. Grapefruit is high in vitamin C; it helps prevent colds and flu, as well as allergic reactions.

Grapes

Another quick-release sugar food and absolutely full of vitamins and nutrients, grapes help to speed up the metabolism and accelerate the elimination of toxins from the body. Melons are another fruit that work in a similar way, actively detoxifying the body. For this reason, these fruits should be eaten alone if possible. Melon makes an excellent first course, speeding the metabolism, as long as you leave at least ten minutes before your main course.

Dates

Containing fructose in such high levels that they are classified as a quick-release food, dates provide an injection of sugar and energy in a "friendly" form. They are also very high in fiber (helping elimination) and mineral rich.

Avocados

A fairly high-fat vegetable, avocados contain essential fat, which is better for the system than saturated fat. Rich in nutrients, they provide energy.

Bananas

A slow-releasing carbohydrate that is very quick to convert to sugar, bananas provide sustained energy over a reasonable period of time and are very high in potassium. Sportsmen and -women eat them to keep up flagging energy levels.

Alfalfa sprouts

The wonder food of the twenty-first century, sprouts are the building blocks of life, and they contain high levels of cleansing chlorophyll. High nutrition in simple form, they form the start of the food chain, containing a huge benefit in a small package!

Seaweed

Seaweed may sound like an unusual foodstuff but the Japanese eat it frequently as part of the delicacy sushi. Seaweed contains iodine, which is important for thyroid function.

Garlic

Several studies confirm that garlic not only has antifungal and antiviral qualities but it also helps to lower high blood pressure, some people even choose to take a garlic oil supplement (make sure you get one that is odor free!) Crushing garlic releases the oil and also beneficial chemical compounds.

Ginger

Warming and uplifting, ginger boosts circulation and is great in cold weather. Drunk as a tea (just chop some gingerroot and infuse in hot water), ginger helps relieve morning sickness for pregnant women, as well as travel sickness. Ginger also aids digestion and stimulates the production of bile.

SPECIAL DIETS

Check with a qualified nutritionist before radically changing your diet, especially with regard to taking vitamin or mineral supplements. The following diets provide an outline only. There has been much research and publicity about the effects of "free radicals" recently. These are imbalanced molecules that have the ability to damage other molecules in the body and have been linked with many ailments from cancer to heart disease. The body naturally fights free radicals with the help of vitamins A, C and E. These are antioxidant nutrients and should have a key role in any balanced diet, but especially for those who are ill, stressed or whose bodies are going through growth or pregnancy.

healthful vitamins and minerals

Pregnancy

Increase folic acid intake by eating lots of vegetables, grains, nuts and seeds. Even the slightest vitamin deficiency in pregnancy can cause problems for the developing baby, so it is well worth seeking dietary advice from a qualified practitioner at this time. Increases of hormone levels (especially a hormone called HCG) can cause "morning sickness," which may in turn affect the nutrients the body can absorb. Try eating little and often, and keep rich, strong foods to a minimum. Foods such as papaya can help balance the hormones, as well as cutting back on dairy products and red meat.

Children

Children need a high-calcium diet, as their bones are still developing. Dairy products can provide this, although in some cases too much dairy in the diet can create eczema and mucus production. Nuts and seeds are also rich in calcium and other minerals, but be careful to grind nuts and seeds for small children.

Healthful balance for busy lifestyles

Even with the best intentions, the hectic lifestyles we lead can mean our diet is often sadly lacking in essential nutrients. Try to take time out to enjoy nutritious food once in a while and not to just view it as fuel to be stocked up on when you feel hungry. Fruit shakes, freshly juiced fruit and vegetables and the occasional "cleanse" can really give your digestive system a boost. Try also to cut down on smoking and alcohol consumption—both of these impair the body's ability to absorb vital nutrients.

Juices

Fresh squeezed fruit and vegetables are one of the most nutritious food types you can consume. Quick to be assimilated and absorbed, they are literally packed with vitamins, minerals and fresh enzymes. Juices cleanse the body from within. Most people find that when they include juices in their diet, they have extra energy, healthier skin, shinier hair, stronger nails and brighter eyes. Most commercially sold juice is made from concentrate and may even contain added sugar, so it is really important to make your own juice from fresh ingredients. There are many juicers on the market at a range of prices, some quite inexpensive.

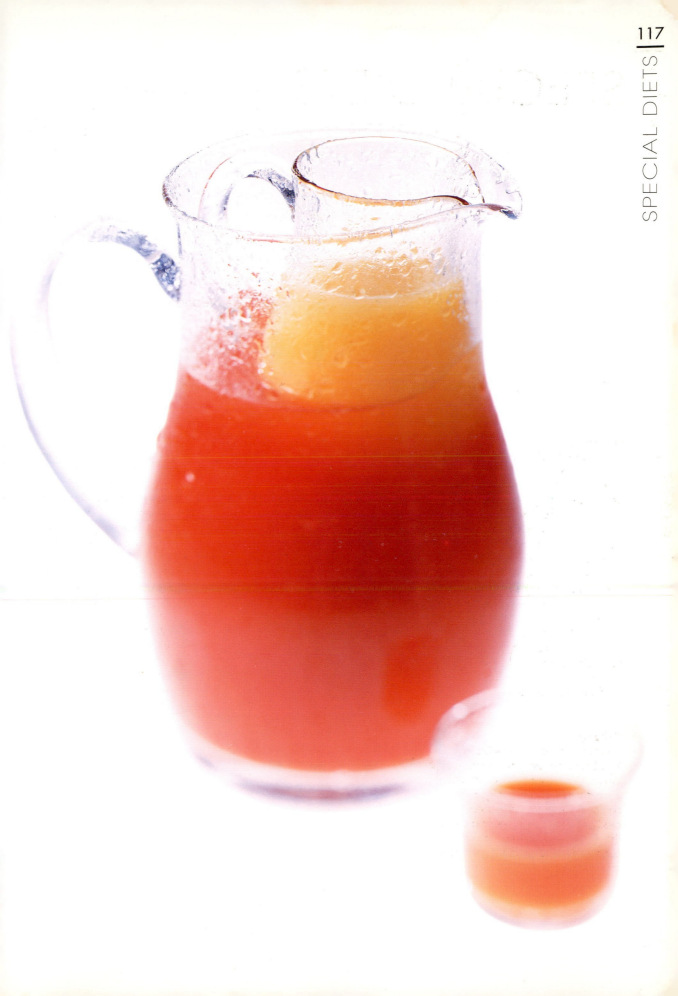

ALLERGIES

The following is a list of ingredients that are potential allergens. They will certainly not provoke an allergic reaction in everyone, and in most cases should only be avoided if you have an allergy you are aware of. Many of the ingredients listed below are much more likely to provoke a reaction if taken internally; it is unusual for any of them to act as an allergen when applied to the skin. All the ingredients used in all the recipes of this book have been selected to be as natural as possible, and no synthetics or preservatives are used. Because of this, most recipes are suitable even for those with extremely sensitive skin.

Milk

Milk contains high amounts of lactose, which some people are allergic to. It may produce rashes or small white pimples under the skin if consumed in large quantities; it may also increase the body's mucus production. When milk is applied to the skin these reactions are much milder than when it is taken internally.

Peanut Oil

A small percentage of the population is highly allergic to peanuts; others are mildly intolerant. Full allergic reaction includes swelling of any area in contact with the peanuts and may even involve swelling and blocking of the body's air passages. A peanut allergy can, in cases such as this, be fatal.

Myrrh

This tincture is worth mentioning briefly as it is very strong and potentially toxic if used in quantities significantly larger than those described in this book. Myrrh is an antifungal and the oil is usually extracted from the gum using solvents; this may also sensitize the skin.

Tea and Green Tea

Both these ingredients contain high amounts of caffeine and tannin, which are strong chemicals that may sensitize the skin. More important, it is a good idea to limit your tea and coffee intake and reduce the levels of caffeine and tannin in your system. Try drinking soothing herbal teas instead. The Chinese use green tea to aid weight loss, as it can stimulate the metabolism.

Cinnamon

This is a strong stimulant, and those with high blood pressure may wish to avoid it.

Lanolin

This is not an allergen, but it may be unsuitable for vegetarians, as it is obtained from sheep's wool and is a slaughterhouse by-product.

Check list of recipes including ingredients listed in allergies section

I suggest using this chart every time you intend to make up a recipe, especially if you are prone to allergic reactions.

Which section is the recipe in?	Which recipe?	Which ingredient is potentially an allergen?
skin	Bran and Oatmeal Scrub p38	milk
	Milk and Rosemary Moisturizer p36	milk
	Myrrh Moisturizer p35	myrrh
	Lime and Peanut Tanning Oil p43	peanut oil
	Lavender and Camomile After-sun Lotion p43	lanolin
hair	Yogurt and Myrrh Conditioner p60	myrrh
eyes	Cucumber Soother p76	tea
	Green Tea Rinse p77	green tea
mouth	Fruit and Nut Lip Salve p82	peanut oil
	Tea Tree, Lavender and Geranium Cold Sore Remedy p82	milk
	Parsley Oil Mouth Rinse p85	milk
	Cinnamon and Calendula Mouthwash p84	cinnamon
	Mandarin Mouthwash p83	milk
bathing	Rose Milk Bath p88	milk
	Honey and Lemon Bath Elixir p88	milk
body Lotions	Camomile and Calendula Dry Skin Cream p97	lanolin
	Rose Moisturizer p96	lanolin
	Apricot Rough Skin Lotion p97	lanolin

BEAUTY PLANNERS

Most of us lead busy lives, and finding time to plan a beauty regimen is not a priority. Perhaps you are used to going to a beauty salon where they will take such concerns off your hands. I find that taking time out to look after my body is a great way of relaxing and caring for myself. It has become a way of life rather than a chore, as has eating healthful food and getting enough sleep. Try to make your beauty regimen part of a habit; get used to coming home at the end of a long day and running a warm bath and lighting a few candles.

This chart should not be followed rigorously, it is meant only to give you some ideas about how to fit natural beauty into your life and adapt it to suit your lifestyle. You will soon find making and using your own preparations is a great way to unwind. If you wish to switch around some of the recipes for certain days; do so according to your skin type. Have fun experimenting!

	Hair	Skin	Nails
Monday	intense conditioning (Jojoba and Vanilla Treatment p57)	cleanse, tone and moisturize as normal	soften the skin of the hands (Apricot Rough Skin Lotion p97)
Tuesday	day of rest; do not wash, just comb through hair gently	exfoliate the skin (Bran and Oatmeal Scrub p38)	remove cuticles (Red Elm Cuticle Softener p67)
Wednesday	wash; do not use styling products	face mask (Grapefruit and Glycerin Mask p24)	moisture treatment (Olive Oil Conditioner p67)
Thursday	hair treatment (Detoxifying Shampoo p55)	problem skin treatment (Fresh Lemon Mask p40)	file and treat your nails (Nail Reviver p67)
Friday	style your hair as normal	normal skin care routine; drink lots of water	color your nails with polish, if you like; use a base coat to protect the nail

This planner provides information for an intense week's treatment for the whole body. Perhaps you can combine it with a week off work, a detoxifying diet or a visit to a health spa. Alternatively, follow part of the plan for targeting specific areas. Use the plan once in a while as an addition to your normal beauty regimen. You can vary the products to fit your skin and hair type. The stages outlined work in sequence, so try to follow the order suggested at least for each body area. For more detailed information on specific areas, for example manicure, see the relevant chapter.

Type of skin condition	What can help?	Cleanse
blemishes	try not to squeeze them! increase your vitamin B intake and zinc if you are female	Orange Sorbet Hot Weather Cleanser p2 or warm water with a drop of tea tree oil
eczema	soak in a warm bath with camomile infused in it	plain aloe vera gel
psoriasis	soak in a warm bath with calendula and chickweed infused in it	Jojoba Two-in-One Cleanser and Moisturiz p27
dry skin (flaky)	soak in a warm bath containing a splash of milk and four drops of palma rosa essential oil	plain aloe vera gel

Problem Skin Chart

Problem skin can be uncomfortable and challenge your self-confidence. Often it is best to treat any problem skin as you would very sensitive skin. Allergies and intolerance to harsh chemical preparations can make any skin condition worse. Try not to bombard your skin with treatments—a simple regimen is best. In severe cases you may wish to visit a practitioner who can address the long-term reasons for your problem skin. Chinese herbalists are especially good.

Dairy products and other mild food intolerance can affect the condition of your skin. Try an elimination diet to identify which specific foods affect you. Simply eliminate one food type at a time from your diet for a week and see how this change affects your skin.

Seek advice from a nutritionist if you are unsure about altering your diet in this way, or if you are unwell or pregnant. Common foods that affect the skin are dairy products, tomatoes, oranges and yeast-rich food.

Tone	Moisturize	Treatment
Lemon Witch Hazel Toner p30	Myrrh Moisturizer p35	Sage and Comfrey Gel p40
Camomile Toner p32	Evening Primrose Moisturizer p41	steam or sauna Tea Tree Face Mask p40
Camomile toner p32 (if needed)	Fresh Lemon Mask p40	steam or sauna Tea Tree Face Mask p40
Rose and Mallow Spritzer p30	Nourishing Orange Oil p34	Banana and Honey Rehydrator p25

Pregnancy

Skin care	During pregnancy your skin can become very itchy and dry, so it is good to moisturize from the beginning of your pregnancy, as a preventative measure. Eczema is an extreme case of this, camomile essential oil in the bath can help. Soften the nipples with cocoa butter to prepare for breast-feeding.
Abdomen	To avoid stretch marks try rubbing wheatgerm oil or vitamin E oil into the abdomen, especially after bathing, to really seal in the moisture. **Massage directly on the stomach is not advised in pregnancy.**
Diet	The most important issue here is making sure you get enough iron in your diet, so eat plenty of leafy green vegetables, or take a supplement. Your eating patterns may change; you may find rather than large meals you prefer to "graze" and eat lightly throughout the day. Keep these snacks healthy—try a handful of nuts or raisins. Keeping well-hydrated can help prevent nausea and tiredness.
Care for your baby	Massage and touch is an important part of making your baby feel loved and connecting with your child. It can help a father to bond with a newly born child.
Care for yourself	Looking after yourself is very important, and many new mothers feel overwhelmed by the responsibility of a young life. Try to take time out and relax when possible.

Yoga and swimming can be of great help throughout your pregnancy to keep you fit and healthy in preparation for the birth.

Raspberry leaf tea, taken in the last few months of your pregnancy, strengthens the uterus ready for childbirth.

Men's Health

he natural body-care industry has long neglected men, although thing are changing, with several forward-thinking companies at the forefront of developments. The fact is that most men are interested in looking after their hair and skin but until recently thought a shower and a shave were enough.

Teenage years	Oily skin and blemishes may be a problem for teenagers. Try to eat a well-balanced diet and cleanse skin carefully and regularly.
Twenties	Most men will need to start shaving during their late teens and early twenties. Do not use a soap-based foam to shave with; a balm is more moisturizing. Wet shaves are generally closer but may leave sensitive skin sore. If you have sensitive skin, use a scented moisturizer after shaving rather than aftershave, which is very astringent. Darker skinned men need to be especially careful to moisturize after shaving to avoid ingrowing hairs, which are painful and may become infected.
Thirties	Moisturizing the skin now helps prevent wrinkles later. Look after your skin and avoid exposure to extremes of temperature and wind over long periods of time.
Mature Skin	Again, moisturizing the skin will help to preserve it. Gentle essential oils such as grapefruit and uplifting rosemary are good for more mature skins. Try using them in the bath: add 4 drops with a splash of whole milk.

Aftershaves are pleasant for any age group, try sandalwood essential oil (diluted in base oil) or Natural Eau de Cologne. Any of the natural recipes in this book can be useful for men, especially shampoos and moisturizers.

INDEX

Acknowledgments

Neal's Yard Remedies
Neal's Yard, Covent Garden
London WC2
Tel: 0171 627 1949

G. Baldwin and Company
FREEPOST LON7690
London SW17 1BR
Tel: 0171 703 5550

Lush
29 High Street, Poole
Dorset BH15 1AB
Tel: 01202 668 545

Culpeper the Herbalist
21 Bruton Street, Berkeley Square
London W1X 7DA
Tel: 0171 629 4559

Gaia Natural Therapies
London Road. Forest Row
East Sussex RH18
Tel: 01342 822 716

South London Natural Health Centre
7a Clapham Common Southside
London SW4 7AA
Tel: 0171 720 4952

The author wishes to thank:
Penny Robinson
Marcus Scott
Pamela Spiers
Alan Spiers
Ali Clark
Julia and Andrew Wright
Robert William
Emily Asher
Rachel Harman
Helen Mundell

Indexer: Dorothy Frame